DizzyClear

Easy to understand dizziness and vertigo and their management, including home treatments.

by

Khalid Bashir

Edited by Mr Jonathan Baker

Grosvenor House
Publishing Limited

This book is published by
Grosvenor House Publishing Ltd
28-30 High Street, Guildford, Surrey, GU1 3EL.
www.grosvenorhousepublishing.co.uk

A CIP record for this book
is available from the British Library

ISBN 978-1-908596-83-3

DIZZYCLEAR

Easy to understand dizziness and vertigo and their management, including home treatments.

Mr Khalid Bashir MD

Consultant and Head of Emergency Medicine Department

Bronglais General Hospital, Aberystwyth, United Kingdom

Specialist in otolaryngology, sports medicine and pre-hospital care

Fellow of College of Emergency Medicine (UK)

Fellow of Royal College of Surgeons (Edinburgh)

Fellow of Royal College of Surgeons (Glasgow)

Diploma in Immediate (pre-hospital) care, Royal College of Surgeons (Edinburgh)

Diploma in Sports Medicine (Cardiff)

Certificate in Aviation Medicine (London)

GMC Specialist register of emergency medicine and general practice

Chapters

Poem

I had dizziness for two years
This brought forth my tears
Someone said it is your ears
Depression was stated by my peers
Stroke was one of my fears
I spent money on pills for years
And then I discovered Dizzyclear
Then my dizziness stopped

By a dizzy patient

Dedication

I would like to dedicate this book to my parents, who have contributed significantly in my life and helped me achieving the highest position in my field.

Acknowledgements

With the help of God and support of my family I was able to complete this book. For this I would like to thank my wife, my lovely daughters and son. Without their help this tremendous task would not have been possible.

Foreword

Doctors and other medical personnel commonly come across patients with dizziness. The incidence of dizziness increases as one gets older. Patients with dizziness can present with and without vertigo sensation. It is quite a disabling symptom, although mostly there is no serious underlying cause. In the past, people suffered and lived with this condition, as care providers found it difficult to deal with it properly; however, with recent advances in technology and proper management of this condition, most people can get very effective treatment. The treatments are usually provided by ear nose and throat specialists, GPs or physiotherapists in the form of various exercises and short term medication.

Dizzyclear has been written by Mr Khalid Bashir, who has vast experience in treating these patients. For the last eleven years, he has successfully treated many patients in Bronglais General Hospital, Aberystwyth. This book also contains many easy to understand illustrations. There is currently a research project being undertaken in this hospital to look into the effectiveness of Epley's manoeuvre and home exercises for the treatment of benign paroxysmal positional vertigo. Initial results have shown significant benefit to these patients in this area of Wales. We feel this book, in simple format and basic structure on this subject, will benefit hospital doctors, GPs, practice nurses, medical students and physiotherapists dealing with dizzy patients on a regular basis.

Dr L Pandya MRCP (UK), MRCP (Ireland), Consultant Physician
Dr M Akram MRCP (UK), Specialty Doctor in Medicine

Important note

Every effort has been made to check the drugs and their doses. The readers are encouraged to consult the drug company's literature before administering any drugs listed in this book. The exercises recommended in this book should be performed in a safe environment, preferably supervised by a clinician or at least in the presence of a relative or a carer.

Directory of Terms

- **BPPV** (Benign paroxysmal positional vertigo). This is a type of dizziness where surroundings appear to spin. It is associated with nausea with various head and neck movements (chapter 23).

- **Dix-Halpike manoeuvre** This is a test for diagnosing BPPV. The head is brought in to various positions to induce dizziness (chapter 26).

- **Proprioception** This is a subconscious sense that enables us to know where our limbs are in space with out having to look. The proprioceptive system consists of nerve receptors in muscles, ligament and tendons around the joints.

- **Nystagmus** A repetitive and involuntary movement of the eyes. If it is present during vertigo diagnostic tests, then the vertigo is very likely due to an inner ear problem.

- **Grommet** A grommet is a small tube inserted into the eardrum, mainly to prevent accumulation of mucus in the middle ear. However, one rare indication of grommet insertion is vertigo due to Meniere's disease.

- **Inner ear** Called *labyrinth* due to its complex shape, the inner ear is situated in the bone behind the ear (petrous part of the temporal bone). It consists of a bony part, called *osseous labyrinth* and a membranous part, called *membranous labyrinth*. The *labyrinth* consists of three parts: 1) *cochlea* is the anterior part of the labyrinth. It is coil-shaped and is responsible for hearing 2) *vestibule* is the central part 3) semi-circular canals are the posterior part of the labyrinth. There are three semi-circular canals named according to their position: superior, posterior and horizontal. The semicircular canals and *vestibule* are concerned with balance.

- **Vestibular system** The part of the inner ear concerned with balance is called the vestibular system. It consists of semi-circular canals and otolith organs. Otolith organs are fluid-filled pouches that lie between the semicircular canals and the cochlea. They are called the utricle and the saccule. These inform the brain when our body is moving in a straight line, such as when standing up or riding in a car. They also inform the brain about the position of our head in relation to the ground, for example, whether we are lying down or sitting

■ **Vestibular rehabilitation therapy (VRT)** This is an exercise-based treatment offered to patients for both acute and chronic dizziness. The following exercises are most commonly used:

• Cooksey-Cawthorne Exercises (chapter 24)
• Gaze Stabilisation Exercises (chapter 25)
• Canalolith repositioning manoeuvres, such as Epley's manoeuvre, Semont's manoeuvre and Brandt Baroff's home exercises (chapters 27&28)

■ **CT scan (Computerised tomogram)** This is a special type of X-ray using a scanner and a computer to take pictures and analyse them. It produces scans in cross-sections. Some scanners are able to turn images into 3-D images.

■ **MRI scan (Magnetic resonance imaging** This is a special type of scan which uses strong magnetic field and radio waves and computers to take and analyse detailed pictures of the brain and spine. It is excellent in differentiating between normal and abnormal soft tissues. There is no radiation exposure to the patient, hence, it is.

Introduction

Do you ever feel dizzy when you get up too quickly, when you change position in the bed, following travel by air, boat or road, or a head injury, or when you turn your head suddenly? You are not alone! Millions of people suffer from dizziness, but few know that effective treatment is available. There are many books available in the market about dizziness that deal with various aspects of dizziness and vertigo. Some of them are difficult to understand by non-medical personnel and others provide much more detail. *Dizzyclear* has been written by an experienced doctor who has successfully treated over 1,100 dizzy patients in the last eleven years. It provides a simple explanation of the causes and symptoms of dizziness and also provides suggestions for relief and self-treatment. *Dizzyclear* will mainly benefit non-specialist medical staff such as GPs, practice nurses, physiotherapists and physical therapists. However, it may also help dizziness and vertigo sufferers.

The book is divided into two parts. The first part of the book covers various causes of dizziness and their management; the second part explains the diagnosis and management of vertigo. Part 2 contains a flow chart which explains how to diagnose and treat vertigo at a GP's surgery or at home. This is supplemented by various easy to understand illustrations.

I used to suffer from recurrent attacks of vertigo for a long time. In spite of being a medic myself and with many of my colleagues being doctors, I did not find any clear, effective treatment. During my training in ear, nose, throat and head and neck surgery, I learned the assessment and treatment of vertigo patients. This helped me significantly in treating my own symptoms. The *Dizzyclear* clinic opened in February 2001, and is based in the Emergency Department of Bronglais Hospital, Aberystwyth, Wales, UK. I am the lead doctor responsible for running this clinic. Patients sometimes refer themselves privately, and we also treat National Health Service patients who are referred by their GP or other specialists.

This clinic was started initially to treat patients suffering from vertigo. However, following successful treatments, we also started seeing patients with dizziness with or without vertigo. We have seen people in our clinic from ages 14 to 94. The duration of symptoms appears to vary from a few months, in the majority, to years, in a few. The longest sufferer was a 60-year-old woman who suffered for nearly 20 years; she was seen in the Dizzyclear clinic. Her symptoms completely settled after a treatment in the clinic (Epley's manoeuvre which involved moving head and neck in some positions) and some days of home exercises. Over 95% of our patients have improved within three weeks of the treatment.

Every effort has been made to provide up to date information in a clear, simple language that is assessable by a wide range of audiences. The first two chapters are dedicated to understanding balance, and how abnormalities in balance can affect our daily life. The remaining chapters cover the wide range of causes of dizziness, providing practical advice for the sufferer, their family members and the relevant health-care professional.

Each chapter begins with a case study outlining the symptoms of real patients; most of them have visited the Dizzyclear clinic over the years. Every effort has been made to disguise the identities of these patients. Following each case study, a brief introduction to each condition is presented, which outlines the symptoms and diagnosis for each condition. This is followed by treatment and advice for health care professional and also for patients. Towards the end there are further reading options which will help if you wish to explore about topics further.

Part 1
Understanding Dizziness and its Management

Chapter 1

What is dizziness?

Dizziness is a feeling that may be hard to describe, and can mean many different things. Some people say that they are "dizzy" when they have light-headedness, or they feel "giddy", or they may experience vertigo or balance problems, or simply feel confused. Vertigo is one very common type of dizziness where you get a sense of movement, or the surroundings appear to spin when you are standing or sitting still. There are various causes of dizziness. Mostly these are minor problems. However, although rare, there could be a serious underlying cause. If you frequently feel dizzy without an obvious cause, then you should see your doctor for further advice.

The exact number of people suffering from dizziness is difficult to quantify, as the diagnostic criteria varies in different places. However, in the United States, from 2001 to 2004, 69 million Americans aged 40 and over were diagnosed with dizziness. The majority of patients over 70 who experience falls have associated dizziness. People with chronic balance problems usually have difficulty in performing one or more daily living tasks, such as bathing, moving about in the house, getting in and out of bed, or dressing.

WHEN TO GET URGENT HELP

You should seek help from your General Practitioner initially, or the nearest emergency department, if you have dizziness along with the following symptoms:

1. Severe headaches, or a different kind of headache than you typically experience
2. High temperature – more than 38°C (100.5°F)
3. Sudden deafness or visual problems such as loss of vision or double vision

4. Weakness or numbness in the body, arm or legs
5. Collapse (passing out)
6. Speech problems
7. Chest pain or a shortness of breath
8. Frequent vomiting (for an hour or more)
9. Irregular pulse rate (i.e. very slow, below 50 bpm, or high, above 100 bpm)
10. Any other concerns

Your doctor would likely examine you and in most cases, there will be clear cause of dizziness after examination. However, sometimes the cause may not be clear and further tests may be required to gain a diagnosis.

CAUSES OF DIZZINESS

Following are the common causes of dizziness. Most causes are discussed in detail in this book:

1. Dizziness due to inner ear problems
- BPPV (benign paroxysmal positional vertigo) – this is the most common cause of dizziness
- Menier's disease
- Vestibular labrynthitis
- Perilymph fistula
- Superior canal dehiscence
- Tumours, such as acoustic neuroma
- Microvascular compression syndrome

2. Dizziness due to neurological problems
- B12 deficiency
- Brain stem strokes
- Basilar invagination
- Epilepsy
- Cervical vertigo
- Chiari malformation
- Migraine associated dizziness

- Motion sickness
- Mal de Debarquement
- Multiple sclerosis
- Parkinson's disease
- Stroke

3. Dizziness due to medical problems
- Low blood pressure
- Side effect of medications

4. Dizziness caused by psychological problems
- Anxiety disorder
- Phobias
- Malingering

5. Dizziness caused by various activities
- Post traumatic dizziness
- Dizziness due to flying
- Motion sickness
- Dizziness due to sexual activity
- Dizziness due to loud sound (Tullio's)
- Positional vertigo

6. Other causes of dizziness
- Post-partum (pregnancy-related)
- Fibromyalgia
- Medication used for epilepsy, high blood pressure, Parkinson's disease, antidepressants, sedatives, and some antibiotics can all cause dizziness

SUMMARY

Dizziness, with or without spinning sensations, is a common complaint. Most causes are simple and easily treatable; however occasionally, there may be a serious underlying illness. With an appropriate examination of a patient's past history and treatment, most people can recover from dizziness. Dizziness has been known to recur, but it can be safely treated at home.

FURTHER READING

1. Agrawal Y, Carey JP, Della Santina CC, Schubert MC, Minor LB. "Disorders of balance and vestibular function in US adults". Arch Intern Med. 200; 169 (10):938-944
2. Neuhauser HK, Radtke A, Von Brevern M, Lezius F, Feldmann M, Lempert T. "Burden of dizziness and vertigo in the community". Arch Intern Med 2008; 168(19): 2118-2124

Chapter 2

How does the balance system work?

Case study: A thirty-five-year old acrobat was referred to a neurology clinic as he had not been able to perform his act of walking on a tight wire for nearly four months. He described a feeling of unsteadiness while practicing his act. This difficulty presented itself after an episode of flu-like illness. His hearing was normal and there were no other concerning sign and symptoms following a thorough examination. He was diagnosed with labrynthitis and was referred for vestibular (inner ear) rehabilitation therapy. Within two months of treatment, he was able to complete his practice session successfully.

The acrobat's vestibular system sends constant signals to the muscles required for this act. The sensory receptors from his eyes, ears, and muscle and joints are constantly sending information to keep him informed of the position of the entire body at every movement. At the same time, the brain is sending signals to the appropriate muscles to contract.

INTRODUCTION

The balance system of our body is quite complex and it is maintained automatically. It does not require conscious control. We only realise when it is not working properly how much we are dependent on this balance system. A balance disorder will make you feel as if you are moving, spinning or floating, even though you are either standing still or lying down. Balance disorders can be caused by various medical conditions involving the inner ear, brain, heart, and lungs, and also as a side effect of certain medications.

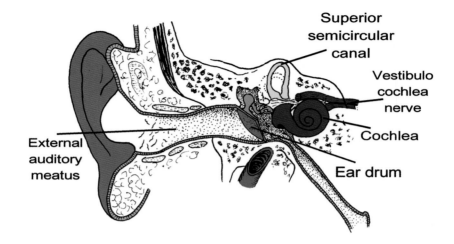

Anatomy of the right ear

Fig 2.1

The ear has two major functions: hearing and balance. The ear is made up of three parts. The outer ear includes the ear canal, the middle ear consists of the eardrum and three tiny bones – the hammer (*malleus*), anvil (*incus*) and stirrup (*stapes*) in accordance with their shapes. Together, they are known as the ossicles. The eustachian tube connects the middle ear to the throat. This helps to equalise the pressure of the middle ear. The inner ear consists of semicircular canals and vestibule for balance and the cochlea for hearing. The sound waves (vibrations) from the environment travel to the eardrum to make it vibrate. These sound vibrations are transferred into mechanical vibrations of the ossicles. This motion is then transferred into electrical impulses sent to the brain via the cochlear nerve.

BALANCE CONTROL

Balance is controlled by the following three systems:

1. Inner ear (vestibular system)

2. Eyes (visual system)
3. Sensory receptors in the skin, muscles and joints maintain our balance when we stand or walk. This is known as proprioception – the body's ability to sense movement

INNER EAR (VESTIBULAR SYSTEM)

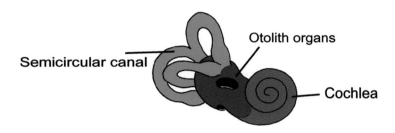

Anatomy of the right labyrinth

Fig 2.2

The part of the inner ear that is concerned with balance is called the vestibular system. This is made up of bones and soft tissue and consists of two parts:

1. Semi-circular canals. These are three fluid-filled channels arranged at right angles to each other. They inform the brain if the head moves in a rotating or circular way e.g. nodding movement and moving the head from left to right.
2. Otolith organs. These are fluid-filled pouches that lie between the semi-circular canals and the cochlea. These inform the brain when our body is moving in a straight line, such as when standing up, or riding in a car. They also inform the brain about the position of our head in relation to the ground – for example, whether we are lying down or sitting. Most of the utricular signals elicit eye movements, while the majority of the saccular signals projects to muscles that control our posture.

MOVEMENTS OF THE HEAD

When the head moves, the fluid inside the semi-circular canals and otolith organs move, too. This movement of fluid causes tiny hairs on the inside lining of both the semi-circular canal and the otolith organs to move. This movement of hair creates a signal that is sent to the brain via a nerve called the vestibular nerve. This conveys information to the brain about the movement and position of the head, even when your eyes are closed.

BALANCE ORGANS WORKING TOGETHER

The vestibular (inner ear) balance organs work well with other balance systems, such as the visual (eyes), and skeletal system (skin, bones and joints) to maintain our balance, both at rest and during motion. The eyes work with the vestibular system to focus on surrounding objects and prevent them from blurring when the head moves, and also keeps us aware of our position when we walk or ride in a car. The position detectors located in the skin, muscles and joints (particularly the neck, ankles, legs and hips) help us maintain our balance when we walk or stand.

FUNCTION OF THE BRAIN IN MAINTAINING BALANCE

The brain uses the most reliable information received from balance organs to control balance. For example, at night the information conveyed by the eyes is reduced, so the brain uses more information from the inner ear, muscles and joints to maintain balance. Whilst walking on sand on a sunny day, the information from feet and joints will be less reliable and the brain will rely more on visuals and the inner ear (vestibular system) to maintain good balance. Therefore, problems with the inner ear balance organs can be compensated for by the eyes, muscle and joint balance receptors.

The brain is fairly good at readjusting to balance problems and after a few days or weeks of balance disorder, most people feel better. However, this process of compensation is not always completely successful, making some individuals feel well on some days and poorly on others. It should be noted that this fluctuation in sensation does not suggest that the problem is getting worse. If you try to carry on your routine activities, this will help the brain to receive the balance information it needs to help it to adapt and recover from this problem. If the recovery process is not complete, then a balance rehabilitation programme would be helpful. This would entail referral to a physical therapist or a physiotherapist by your GP or ear, nose and throat specialist.

SUMMARY

Maintaining balance is a function of different parts of the body. They work together in a very smooth manner. Occasionally, when one of the systems is not working, we become unsteady. The brain tends to compensate and help in recovery. Sometimes the patient may need to be referred to a therapist for vestibular rehabilitation therapy, which is an exercise programme to help in recovery.

Chapter 3

Meniere's disease and dizziness

Case study: A fifty-year old schoolteacher attended the Dizzyclear clinic with three months' history of fluctuating hearing loss and vertigo episodes. These attacks were getting more frequent, and lasting up to two days on occasion. During these episodes, she often had to stay in bed, which led to her having to take many days off work. She also noted "fullness in the ear" and weak legs during these episodes. On one occasion, she called her GP for a home visit, who administered an intramuscular injection for sickness and dizziness, which improved her symptoms. Her mother wears a hearing aid and her symptoms started like this, but left her with permanent deafness. All examinations were normal, and the patient was started on medications for Meniere's disease. She was followed up at three months with very good progress.

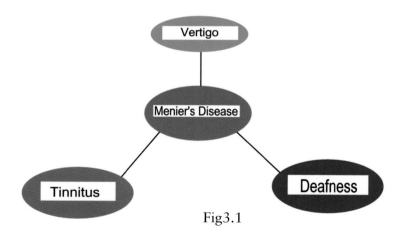

Fig3.1

INTRODUCTION

Meniere's disease is a progressive disease of the inner ear, which damages both the hearing and the balance part of inner ear. It usually starts in one ear and with time, can involve both ears. It can occur at any age. However, it typically presents in people between the ages of 20 to 50.

CAUSE & SYMPTOMS

There is no single known cause for this condition. However, it is thought to be caused by increased pressure of fluid in the inner ear (membranous labyrinth). This increased pressure may cause leakage of fluid between different parts of the labyrinth. This process may cause the inner ear to send confusing messages to the brain, resulting in dizziness and vomiting. It is possible that more fluid (endolymp) is produced than absorbed in the inner ear, leading to increased pressure.

Risk factors

1. Genetic link: there is usually a family history of Meniere's disease
2. Metabolic disturbance leading to sodium and potassium imbalance (salt imbalance)
3. Viral infections including meningitis can cause the impairment of absorption of fluid from the inner ear, leading to symptoms of Meniere's disease
4. Immune system abnormality, where antibodies start attacking the body's own tissues, leading to abnormal fluid absorption
5. High salt intake, increased coffee, alcohol, nicotine, stress, monosodium glutamate and various allergies have all been reported as triggers for Meniere's disease
6. Side effects of some medicines can produce similar symptoms to Meniere's disease, for instance, anticonvulsants, antidepressants, sedatives, antihistamines and antipsychotics

Normal pure-tone audiogram

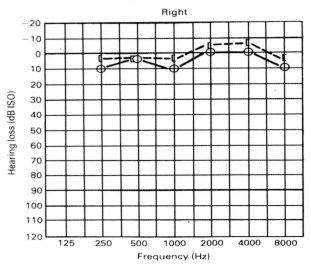

Fig 3.2.

Audio-gram showing sensorineural deafness

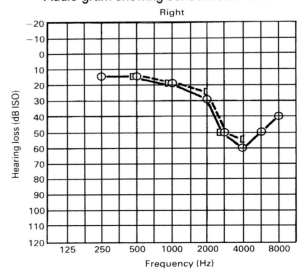

Fig 3.3.

The symptoms of Meniere's disease include the following:

1. Vertigo (episodic spinning sensation)
2. Deafness (degree of hearing loss is variable – initially, it is intermittent, then usually progresses to permanent loss)
3. Tinnitus. This is characteristically low pitch (like listening to a seashell or machinery)
4. Ear pressure, which feels like ear fullness
5. It may also cause increase stress, anxiety and depression
6. Sensations of disequilibrium or dizziness

The duration of symptoms varies from minutes to hours, and can be quite sporadic, with symptom-free periods of months and years in between the attacks. Some people collapse during the attacks. These drop attacks are not common, but quite frightening, as they can come without any warning. Many individuals can become quite tired after an acute attack.

DIAGNOSIS & TREATMENT

There is no specific test to diagnose Meniere's disease. The diagnosis is usually made with history, examination and an audiogram (a hearing test). This hearing test may return normal results, or may show deafness in one or both ears (sensorineural deafness). Occasionally, a brain scan is undertaken to rule out other causes such as stroke, tumour and bleeding. A relatively new test called vestibular evoked myogenic potential is being used, and this can show some specific changes for diagnosis and also for monitoring of the condition. The American Academy of Otolaryngology and Head and Neck Surgery has established criteria to diagnose Meniere's disease, which include the following:

1. Two spontaneous episodes of rotational vertigo lasting at least 20 minutes
2. Sensorineural hearing loss confirmed on a hearing test
3. Tinnitus and/or a perception of aural fullness

Treatment of acute attacks of Meniere's disease

1. Medications called vestibular sedatives and antiemetics are given in an acute attack. Prochlorperazine and Cinnarizine are used for nausea, vomiting and dizziness.
2. Diazepam or lorazepam in small doses and for a short period will help to improve the symptoms.
3. Intravenous fluids may be needed if there is a risk of dehydration.

Treatment of chronic attacks and prevention of Meniere's disease

If the attacks are less frequent and mild in nature, then you may not need any further medication. If the mild symptoms return, then the above treatment should be sufficient. However, if the attacks are frequent and severe, you may need further treatment.

Medical treatment

1. Betahistine hydrochloride is considered to be helpful in disease prevention. It improves the blood supply to the inner ear, hence increasing the absorption of fluid, leading to decreased pressure in the labyrinth (inner ear). It is usually taken for 3-6 months before real benefit is achieved.
2. Diuretics and beta-blockers have reported some success in chronic treatment by reducing the fluid pressure in the inner ear.
3. Vestibular rehabilitation therapy is particularly good for patients who have responded to medical or surgical treatment but still have some residual symptoms of disequilibrium.

Surgical treatment

1. The destructive procedure includes intratympanic gentamicin injection, labyrinthectomy, and vestibular nerve section. Destructive procedures are tried when medical treatment has failed. These procedures are associated with a high incidence of hearing loss.

2. The non-destructive procedures include endolymphatic sac decompression and sacculotomy. These procedures are associated with a low risk of sensorineural hearing loss and are commonly performed in patients with normal hearing

ADVICE FOR HEALTH-CARE PROFESSIONALS

1. Other possible causes that can present with symptoms similar to Meniere's disease include neurofibromatosis, multiple sclerosis, migraine, diabetes, thyroid disease and transient ischemiac attack.
2. Hearing aids may be needed if the deafness is worse in both ears.
3. Patients have reported improvement in their symptoms after taking herbal medicines and multivitamins, but there is no robust scientific evidence to support this treatment.
4. If tinnitus is a real problem in patients, they can be referred for tinnitus rehabilitation therapy.

ADVICE FOR PATIENTS & CARERS

1. During an acute attack, lie down with your eyes focused on a distant object. If possible, you should stay in this posture until the attack subsides.
2. Inform your friends and family members about this condition so they can help you during an acute attack.
3. About 90-95% of patient with Meniere's disease are able to live normally.
4. Lifestyle adjustments, including avoidance of the above trigger factors, are usually required.
5. Salt restriction to 2-3 G per day is appropriate. Caffeine and nicotine are vasoconstrictors that may cause decreased blood supply to the inner ear. Alcohol may cause fluid and salt imbalance. Hence, you should limit yourself to one cup of coffee and one alcoholic drink per day.
6. Try and avoid heights, ladders and swimming alone.
7. There are driving restrictions if you are diagnosed with Meniere's disease.

8. Make sure that appropriate safety steps been considered at home as the attacks can happen any time without warning. For instance, you may want a railing to hold in the toilet, and along the staircase and bedroom – and make sure any sharp edges, such as radiators, are covered. Further help and support is available from various charities such as www.meniers.org.uk and www.tinnitus.org.uk.

SUMMARY

Meniere's sufferers usually have a history of fluctuating deafness, episodic vertigo, aural fullness and tinnitus. It is a life-altering disease. Most people are able to live a normal life with the help of lifestyle adjustment and medication. About 10% of patients may need surgical treatment at some time during this illness.

FURTHER READING

1. Kinney, SE, Sandridge SA, Newman CW. "Long-term effects of Meniere's disease on hearing and quality of life". Am J Otol 1997 Jan; 18 (1): 67-73
2. Klockars, T, Kentala, E. "Inheritance of Meniere's disease in the Finnish population". Arch Otolaryngol Head Neck Surg 2007; 133:73
3. Anderson JP, Harris JP. "Impact of Meniere's disease on quality of life". Otol Neurotol 22:888-894, 2001
4. Perez-Garrigues, H, Lopez-Escamez, JA, Perez, P, et al. "Time course of episodes of definitive vertigo in Meniere's disease". Arch Otolaryngol Head Neck Surg 2008; 134:1149
5. Committee on Hearing and Equilibrium guidelines for the diagnosis and evaluation of therapy in Meniere's disease. American Academy of Otolaryngology Head and Neck Foundation, Icn. Otolaryngology Head Neck Surg 1995; 113:181.

Chapter 4

Vestibular Neuritis (Labyrinthitis) and dizziness

Case study: A paramedic brought a fifty-year-old to the emergency department suffering from intense episodes of dizziness and vomiting over a 12-hour period. He called for an ambulance as he felt unable to cope with his symptoms, which he reported as a feeling of tiredness and vomiting every time he moved out of bed. After a careful history and an examination, he was diagnosed with labyrinthitis. He was given an injection (prochlorperazine) for vomiting and dizziness. After about four hours, he began to feel better, but was kept in the hospital overnight for observation, and discharged the next day.

INTRODUCTION

Vestibular neuritis, also called labyrinthitis, is a benign, self-limiting condition affecting one, or both, inner ears. The term vestibular neuritis is generally used when only the vestibular nerve is affected (balance), whereas labyrinthitis is used where both the vestibular nerve and labyrinth (hearing and balance) are involved. The symptoms can be disabling for short periods of time, but appear to be temporary, as most people recover following treatment.

CAUSES & SYMPTOMS

The exact cause of labyrinthitis is unknown. However, there are a few possible causes:

1. Viral infection. Almost 50% of people have cold or flu before developing labyrinthitis. The herpes zoster (chickenpox) and mumps virus are also thought to cause this condition.
2. Bacterial infection. Bacteria that cause middle ear infection, meningitis and mastoiditis can travel to the labyrinth (inner ear) to cause infection. Bacterial infections are generally considered more serious than viral infections.

3. Autoimmune conditions. The body's immune system produces antibodies to fight infection. However, with autoimmune conditions, they may start attacking their own healthy tissue like the labyrinth, leading to inflammation and labyrinthitis.

There are a few known risk factors that encourage the development of labyrinthitis:

- Recent history of "cold" symptoms, with temperature, aches and pains, coughs, tiredness etc
- Contact with someone with similar symptoms
- Migraine
- Diabetes
- Recent ear operation
- Recent trauma
- Medications, including those for epilepsy, ear infections, and some tranquilisers

Symptoms vary between individuals. Severe symptoms may last for 1-2 days, but mild symptoms can last for a few weeks and include:

- Vertigo
- Tinnitus
- Deafness
- Earache
- Ear discharge when the underlying cause is infection
- High temperature: 38 degrees C or above
- Nystagmus (involuntary movements of the eyes)
- Skin blisters, if the shingles virus is the underlying cause
- Vomiting and nausea
- Sore throat, cough and painful neck muscles
- Red eye or blurring of vision

DIAGNOSIS & TREATMENT

This condition is usually diagnosed after a detailed check of the patient's history and a clinical examination. There is no single confirmatory test available for this condition. However, severe symptoms and no response to treatment would indicate that further tests may be required. These include:

- Hearing test to look for hearing loss (sensorineural deafness)
- Balance test to asses vestibular functions
- Blood test to exclude any infection
- Brain scans to check if there is any cause in the brain causing these symptoms, such as stroke

Mild symptoms can be treated at home. However if symptoms are severe then hospital treatment may be needed. Disease-specific treatment includes the following:

1. Corticosteroid use in the acute stage has been shown to improve in early recovery.
2. Antiviral agents like acyclovir have been shown to improve symptoms in some patients, although these are not widely used.
3. Other treatments include anti-sickness medications such as prochlorperazine. Sedatives like diazepam will help with relaxation and sleep.
4. Surgical treatment is occasionally needed to drain the infection in the middle and inner ear (mastoidectomy).
5. Vestibular rehabilitation therapy is an exercise-based programme that improves brains ability in improving balance.

ADVICE FOR HEALTH-CARE PROFESSIONALS

1. Consider the possibility of a stroke (cerebellum and brainstem infarction) if symptoms are severe and the patient does not respond to therapy. This may require magnetic resonance imaging (MRI) or an angiography (MRA) to confirm the diagnosis.
2. Other conditions to consider are meningitis, Meniere's disease, multiple sclerosis, tumours of the brain, arthritis of the neck (cervical spondylosis), and migrainous vertigo.
3. Medications are usually taken for 48 hours, as prolonged treatment may impair the brain's compensation response and delay complete recovery.

4. Early start of vestibular rehabilitation therapy improves balance in the long term.
5. In a small number of patients, the symptoms can persist for months and even years.

ADVICE FOR PATIENTS & CARERS

1. During an acute attack, a sufferer should lie still with their eyes closed until symptoms improve.
2. Rest and sleep can help to improve the symptoms.
3. Consult your GP if the symptoms are severe or if they are not better with 48 hours.
4. Do not drive or operate machinery when suffering from acute symptoms.

SUMMARY

Vestibular neuritis or acute labyrinthitis is usually caused by a virus and presents with vertigo, nausea, and vomiting and gait abnormality. Diagnosis can be made by a review of the patient's history and an examination, without the need for investigations. Early treatment with medications and vestibular rehabilitation therapy improves long-term recovery. Most acute symptoms get better within 1-2 days. However, mild symptoms can last for weeks.

FURTHER READING

1. Strupp, M, Zingler, VC, Arbusow, V, et al. "Methyprednisole, Valacyclovir, or the combination for vestibular neuritis". N Engl J Med 2004; 351:351
2. Baloh, RW. "Clinical practice. Vestibular neuritis". N Engl J Med 2003; 348:1027
3. Hotson, JR, Baloh, RW. "Acute vestibular syndrome". N Engl J Med 1998; 339:680

Chapter 5

Perilymphatic fistula (PF) and dizziness

Case study: A forty-five-year-old man was suffering from imbalance and intermittent deafness following ear surgery performed four years before. Whilst living in the countryside, he had learned to cope with these symptoms. However, since moving to London, his symptoms had got worse. This appears to coincide with travelling on the underground and using lifts more frequently. He also noted that whilst exercising in the gym with heavy weights, the symptoms would recur again. He was initially diagnosed with Meniere's disease, but the treatment offered did not help. His doctor then referred him to see an ear, nose and throat specialist. After careful examination and following various tests, he was diagnosed with PF. He was advised to use three pillows at night, to avoid lifting weights in the gym, and where possible, to use alternative transport rather than the underground. He returned to his doctor for his four-week follow up, and reported that his symptoms had improved, and so no further treatment was offered. He was given an option to have surgery if the problem recurred or if his symptoms got worse.

INTRODUCTION

PF is an abnormal communication between the air-filled middle ear and the fluid-filled inner ear. Normally, the inner ear fluid is contained in the rigid bones but with PF, this can leak into the middle ear. PF may lead to intermittent vertigo associated with fluctuating hearing loss. Flying can make symptoms worse due to change in the pressure in the inner ear. The signs and symptoms are usually similar to those of Meniere's disease.

CAUSES & SYMPTOMS

1. Trauma is the most common cause (usually from a direct injury/blow to the ear).

2. Following an ear surgery e.g. stapedectomy – an operation to correct deafness (called otosclorsis) by removing the middle ear bone (stapes)
3. Chronic ear infections such as cholesteatoma can cause PF
4. Congenital (present since birth). PF should be suspected in children with a recurrent history of meningitis. It is possible that they have a congenital abnormality of the middle or inner ear.

Symptoms
- Dizziness and imbalance
- Vertigo
- Nausea and vomiting
- Fullness and increased pressure in the ears
- Deafness or partial hearing loss, usually fluctuating in nature
- Tullio's phenomenon, in which symptoms of dizziness get worse on exposure to a loud noise
- Activities like coughing, sneezing, lifting and straining may make symptoms worse
- Disorganisation of memory and concentration
- Tinnitus may be roaring in nature

Activities that trigger symptoms of PF
- Forceful nose blowing
- Straining due to constipation or prostate problems
- Lifting heavy objects
- Scuba diving can cause large changes in the atmospheric pressure and pressure in the head, particularly in rapid ascent
- Bending over
- Air travel can cause pressure changes, particularly in small, unpressurised planes, and this can lead to the development of PF
- Using escalators and lifts, especially those travelling at high speed, can increase symptoms
- Loud noise of music or instruments

DIAGNOSIS & TREATMENT

It is not easy to diagnose PF. However, the following tests are usually helpful:

1. Fistula test. This test is performed by applying pressure in the ear canal, either by pressing the tragus or by using pneumatic otoscope. The positive test is associated with nystagmus (involuntary movements of the eyes).
2. Positive pressure (Valsalva's manoeuvre). Forced expiration with pinched nostrils may induce symptoms of PF.
3. Hearing test. This may show deafness on the diseased side (sensorineural deafness).
4. Magnetic resonances imaging (MRI) scan or computerised tomogram (CT scan) of the brain are usually helpful to exclude other causes such as infection or tumours.
5. Endoscopic examination. This test will definitely confirm the fistula. It is performed by using a small endoscope (camera), introduced through the ear canal towards the inner ear.

Non-surgical treatment:

This is most commonly used. Strict bed rest for about one week is advised, followed by avoidance of the activities that made the symptoms worse. It can take up to six months for fistula to heal.

Surgical treatment:

If the PF does not heal, usually after six months, or if the symptoms are very severe, then surgical treatment is offered. The surgical treatment depends upon the location of the fistula.

ADVICE FOR HEALTH-CARE PROFESSIONALS

1. With severe symptoms, always consider the possibility of Meniere's disease, stroke, or acoustic neuroma.
2. If there are associated symptoms of a "cold", like blocked sinuses and eustachian tubes, then a decongestant spray or decongestant medication may help.
3. Tranquilisers such as diazepam or lorazepam may help some individuals.

4. Air travel is not recommended, as pressure changes can make the symptoms worse. If air travel is unavoidable, then nasal decongestant spray and earplugs may help. Rarely, ventilation tubes (grommets) are used to prevent the symptoms during air travel.
5. Most patients get better by sleeping on pillows propped up at about 30 degrees, and by avoiding the trigger factors

ADVICE FOR PATIENTS

1. The symptoms can get worse while shopping in a supermarket, particularly going up and down aisles, so take someone with you for assistance until symptoms are improve.
2. Take special care while walking at night. Make sure that hallways at home are free of obstruction, as you may lose your balance and risk a fall or other injury. If needed, you can use a walking stick. Don't drive a car at night and in stormy weather, as decreased visibility will make your balance worse.
3. Modification of daily activities is necessary to cope with this problem, particularly avoiding the trigger factors.

SUMMARY

Perilymphatic fistula is a rare condition where abnormal communication develops between the inner and middle ear, leading to a hearing loss, tinnitus, vertigo and dizziness. There are still controversies surrounding diagnosis and treatment. Most commonly it is treated with rest, and by avoiding trigger factors. Modifications in lifestyle are needed to cope with the symptoms.

FURTHER READING

1. Hakuba, N, Hato N, Sinomori, Y, Sato H, Goto K. "Labyrinthine fistula as a late complication of middle ear surgery using the canal wall down technique". Otol Neurotol 23:832-835,2002

2. Fuse T, Tada, Y, Aoyagi, M, Sugai Y. "CT detection of facial canal dehiscence and semicircular canal fistula: comparison with surgical findings". J of computer assisted tomograpghy 20(2): 221-4,1996
3. Hain, TC, Ostrowski, VB. "Limits of normal pressure sensitivity in the fistula test". Audiology and Neuro-otology 2:384-390, 1997
4. Kokker, M, Vesterhauge, S. "Perilyphatic fistula in cabin attendants: an incapacitating consequence of flying with a common cold". Aviat Space Environ Med. 2005; 76(1):66-8

Chapter 6

Vitamin B12 deficiency and dizziness

Case study: A 75-year-old woman reported feelings of dizziness, vague abdominal pains and generalised weakness to her GP and informed him that she had felt this way for the last year or so. The doctor undertook a thorough examination, blood tests, an audiometric evaluation (hearing test) and a scan of her brain. These tests revealed that she was suffering from anaemia and had particularly low levels of Vitamin B12. Following a course of Vitamin B12 supplementation, her symptoms improved, and with time, vanished.

INTRODUCTION

Vitamin B12, also called cobalamin, is needed for red blood cell production and normal functioning of the nerve cells. Vitamin B12 deficiency can cause nerve damage, which is called "B12 neuropathy". This neuropathy may lead to tingling, numbness, and weakness of the legs and arms. Patients with Vitamin B12 deficiency have difficulty in identifying the position of their arm and legs (loss of position sense). This loss of position sense usually leads to dizziness. Some people may develop confusion, depression, decreased mental function and dementia.

A clear perception of vitamin B12 absorption will help to understand the causes of deficiency. Vitamin B12 cannot be absorbed on its own and requires an acidic environment within the stomach to break down and be absorbed. This process is aided by a protein called intrinsic factor (IF), which is produced in the stomach (parietal) cells and binds to Vitamin B12 in the duodenum (upper small intestine). This vitamin B12-intrinsic factor complex subsequently aids in the absorption of vitamin B12 in the terminal ileum (lower small intestine). Vegans can become deficient, as Vitamin B12 is naturally found in animal products such as milk, meat, and eggs.

CAUSES & SYMPTOMS

Some common causes include:

- Pernicious anaemia (lack of absorption of Vitamin B12 due to deficiency of intrinsic factor)
- Inadequate diet
- Increased need e.g. in children and during pregnancy
- Defective absorption from the intestine
- Surgical removal of part of the stomach
- Certain drugs can may affect the absorption of Vitamin B12, such as metformin (for diabetes), colchicine (for gout), antacids and some anti-epilepsy drugs

This disease is largely asymptomatic, but in some, it can present with following symptoms:

- Tiredness (due to anaemia)
- Pale skin, often with a lemon tint
- Breathless after little exertion
- Palpitations and headaches
- Unsteady gait (sensory ataxia) with loss of position sense
- When associated with spinal cord, it is called "sub-acute combined degeneration"
- Weakness and numbness in hands and feet
- Increased risk of osteoporosis, leading to hip and spine fracture
- Sore mouth and tongue
- Poor resistance to infections
- Dementia and other neurological symptoms

DIAGNOSIS & TREATMENT

1. A blood test is usually undertaken to diagnose deficiency of Vitamin B12. Serum blood levels of Vitamin B12 may be low (normal >190ng/l).
2. A special test called a Schilling test is done to discern whether the cause is dietary or due to malabsorption.

3. Brain scans may show abnormalities of the white matter of the brain or spine.
4. Nerve conduction studies may show abnormalities (axonal dysfunction).

If treatment is started early (within two months of onset), there is a good chance of complete recovery. However, if it is not treated, the disease may progress further and the patient may become bed-bound.

ADVICE FOR HEALTH-CARE PROFESSIONALS

1. Consider treatment if Vitamin B12 levels are low (less than 130ng/l). It is mostly given in injection form.
2. B12 deficiency usually requires lifelong monitoring.
3. If folic acid is given alone, it will improve the blood picture, but may cause irreversible neurological damage.

ADVICE FOR PATIENTS & CARERS

1. You only need a small amount if Vitamin B12 daily (1.5 micrograms). In otherwise healthy individuals, a balanced diet will provide this, and you are unlikely to have a shortage.
2. Vitamin B12 can be taken in healthy individuals in oral tablets, usually available in combination with other supplements from pharmacies and health shops.
3. Natural food sources of Vitamin B12 include meat, fish, poultry, and eggs.
4. If you eat a vegan diet, it is possible that you may develop a deficiency, as B12 is not found in fruits, vegetables and grains. Consider Vitamin B12-fortified foods in your diet, such as fortified breakfast cereals or cereal bars.

SUMMARY

Vitamin B12 deficiency is a rare cause of dizziness. It is usually investigated when there is no other cause of dizziness found. It is important to get early treatment, as the symptoms resolve completely with successful treatment.

FURTHER READING

1. Butler CC, Vidal-Alaball J, Cannings-John, R, et al. "Oral vitamin B12 versus intramuscular vitamin B12 for vitamin B12 deficiency: a systemic review of randomised controlled trials". Fam Pract 2006; 23:279-285
2. Stone, KL, Bauer, DC, Sellmeyer, D, Cummings, SR. "Low serum vitamin B12 levels are associated with increased hip-bone loss in older women: a prospective study". J Clin Endocrinol Metab 2004; 89:1217
3. Cagacci, A, Baldassari, F, Rivolta, G, et al. "Relation of homocystine, folate, and vitamin B12 to bone mineral density of postmenopausal women". Bone 2003; 22:956
4. Tangeney, C and others. "Biochemical indicators of vitamin B12 and folate insufficiency and cognitive" Neurology 2009:72: 361-367

Chapter 7

Motion sickness

Case study: A seven-year-old was seen in the Dizzyclear clinic with a two-year history of being a "poor traveller". She used to get excessively "sick" on journeys. Family trips would be disturbed due to her constant travel sickness. She was otherwise in a good health, and was not taking any regular medication. An examination by her GP showed no obvious cause of her symptoms. She was given medicine for travel sickness to start 6-8 hours before the journey and advice regarding the prevention of motion sickness. For the first time, she was able to complete her journey without any vomiting and stops.

INTRODUCTION

Motion sickness is an unpleasant condition which is characterized by nausea, dizziness and vomiting. It occurs when the balance is affected by motion. It is sometimes referred to as carsickness, seasickness, or airsickness due to the mode of travel. Motion sickness is much more common in children, and it can be prevented by medications. Although it is uncomfortable, it is not serious. It is not clearly understood why only some people develop motion sickness. Symptoms usually stop when the journey is over. However, in some people, it may last for a few hours and on occasion, sometimes days after the journey.

CAUSES & SYMPTOMS

Motion sickness is caused by a discrepancy between what you see and what you feel. Normally, the brain receives balance signals from the inner ear (gravity and acceleration), eyes (vision), and various parts of the body, including joints, muscle and skin sensors/receptors (proprioception). When there is an intentional motion, such as walking, all of the three signals are interpreted appropriately without any conflict. However, in an unusual motion, such as travelling in a car, train, boat or even watching a movie, the eyes tell the brain that there is movement, but the inner ear and proprioception tells the brain that there is no movement, which results in conflicting information.

Example 1. If a person is sitting inside the cabin of a ship, his eyes send signals to the brain that the surroundings are not moving. However, due to the movement of the ship, both vestibular systems and proprioception send signals to the brain that surroundings are moving. These conflicting signals cause motion sickness.

Example 2. If a person is watching a movie or playing a game, particularly on a large screen, the eyes will send a signal to the brain that the surroundings are moving. But as there is no physical movement, both the vestibular system and proprioception will send signals to the brain that the surroundings are not moving, so this conflicting signal will cause motion sickness.

Vestibular signals are very important in the occurrence of motion sickness, as animals with no or inactivated inner ears do not develop motion sickness. However, visual signals are less important in the development of this condition, as blind subjects as well as persons with normal vision develop the same symptoms of motion sickness. Motion sickness gets better with repeated exposure to the provoking stimuli, as has been observed in pilots with almost 50% symptoms in the first flight and about 24% in subsequent flights.

The symptoms are variable in different people. Common symptoms are described below:

- Sweating
- Drooling
- Nausea and vomiting
- Headaches
- Pale appearance, which may lead to fainting

- Feeling cold and shaking
- Belching
- Tiredness
- Hyperventilation may lead to numbness of fingers, shortness of breath and feeling of impending doom

DIAGNOSIS & TREATMENT

A number of medications are available, both on prescription from a GP and from pharmacies. Prevention treatments are more effective than actually treating the symptoms.

1. Antihistamine. There are a number of preparations available for treating motion sickness. These include chlorpheniramine, cyclizine, cinnarizine and meclizine (in the USA).
2. Benzodiazepines like diazepam and lorazepam may be useful.
3. Hyosine hydrobromide (Scopolamine) is commonly used mainly for the prevention of motion sickness. It is available in various pharmacies without prescription. It comes in various forms, including tablets and patches.
4. Promethazine is an antidopaminergic usually taken the night before travel, available through a prescription by GP.

ADVICE FOR HEALTH-CARE PROFESSIONALS

1. Children can be safely given medications for prevention of motion sickness, e.g. cinnarizine, also available over the counter.
2. Pregnant patients are more prone to motion sickness. Prochlorperazine is felt to be safe to be used for this condition.
3. The Puma method consists of conditioning exercises and claims to prevent motion sickness.

ADVICE FOR PATIENTS & CARERS

1. Avoid heavy meals and drinks, as these may worsen motion sickness.

2. Try and sit where there is least motion, e.g. lower level cabins near the centre of ship, over the wing in an aeroplane and at the front of a car.
3. Avoid reading if you are prone to motion sickness.
4. Acupressure can be helpful: apply gentle pressure about one inch above the wrist joint between the two tendons or a wrist.
5. Take short breaks on longer journeys to have oral fluids, fresh air, and walk about.
6. Open a window or vent for fresh air.
7. If nausea starts, try and breathe deeply while focusing on a distant object.
8. Ginger can improve nausea. It can be taken as a drink or biscuits.
9. Separate yourself from others suffering from motion sickness. This appears to have some psychological effect on reducing symptoms.
10. Sleeping during the journey may help to prevent or relieve symptoms.

SUMMARY

Motion or travel sickness is very common and can make you feel sick or vomit. It is caused by repeated unusual movements, usually when travelling by car, boat, plane or train. There are effective treatments available, both from your doctor and the pharmacist. Ideally, medicines should be taken before the journey is started.

FURTHER READING

1. Brizzee, KR, Igarashi, M. "Effect of macular ablation on frequency and latency of motion-induced emesis in the squirrel monkey". Aviat Space Environ Med 1986; 57:1066
2. Miller EF, 2nd, Graybiel, A. "Semi-circular canals as a primary stiological factor in motion sickness". Aerosp Med 1972; 43:1065

3. Nicholson, AN, Stone, BM, Turner, C, Mills, SL. "Central effects of cinnarizine: restricted use in aircrew". Aviat Space Environ Med 2002; 73:570

4. Cowings, PS, Toscano, WB, DeRoshia, C, Miller, NE. "Promethazine as a motion sickness treatment: impact on human performance and mood states". Aviat Space Environ Med 2000; 71:1013

5. Gordon, CR, Gonen, A, Nachum, Z, et al. "The effects of dimenhydrinate, cinnarizine and transdermal scopolamine on performance". J Psychopharmacol 2001; 15:167

6. Hu, S, Stritzel, R, Chandler, A, Stem, RM. "P6 acupressure reduces symptoms of vection-induced motion sickness". Aviat Space Environ Med 1995; 66:631

Chapter 8

Mal de Debarquement Syndrome (MDS)

Case study of MDS: A 55-year-old woman reported a feeling of unsteadiness, and described her symptoms as "trying to walk on a mattress or trampoline" to her GP after returning home from a cruise. The examination by the doctor was unremarkable and medication had no effect. The condition was explained to her, and her symptoms improved in the following three months with the help of home exercises. She was able to cope better with the help of home exercises.

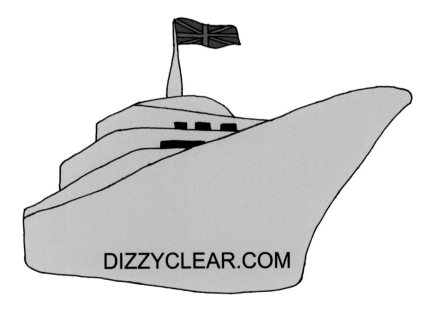

Fig 8.0

INTRODUCTION

The term Mal de Debarquement comes from a French phrase which, when roughly translated, means "disembarkation sickness." It is an imbalance or rocking sensation which is often both "felt" and ""seen" by the sufferer and typically occurs after exposure to motion (such as a sea cruise, flight or road journey). The cause of this condition is most likely present in the balance areas of the brain, rather than the inner ear. The brain adapts to this motion by sending signals to the co-ordination muscles, which help in adjusting to the environment. This adaptation is like developing "sea legs". On cessation of this journey, the brain should develop "land legs" to adapt to the land environment, but in some individuals fails to do so and the illusion of movement persists. Most individuals (90%) who develop MDS are women in their 50s and 60s.

A well-known reference to the syndrome was made by Erasmus Darwin, in 1796. He wrote: "Those who have been upon the water in a boat or ship so long, that they have acquired the necessary habits of motion upon that unstable element, at their return on land frequently think in their reveries, or between sleeping and waking, that they observe the room, they sit in, or some of its furniture, to liberate like the motion of the vessel. This I have experienced myself, and have been told, that after long voyages, it is some time before these ideas entirely vanish. The same is observable in a less degree after having travelled some days in a stage coach, and particularly when we lie down in bed, and compose ourselves to sleep; in this case it is observable, that the rattling noise of the coach, as well as the undulatory motion, haunts us."

CAUSES & SYMPTOMS

The exact cause of this condition is currently unclear; however experts suggest a number of possible explanations:

- MDS is linked with problems in the balance organ in the brain, rather than the inner ear
- MDS is a variant of migraine, as most patients also suffer headaches

- As the condition largely occurs in females, it may be linked to sex hormones, such as oestrogen or progesterone
- It could also be genetic, related to two copies of the X chromosome, perhaps combined with other susceptibility factors
- It may be caused by the Norwalk virus, which is common on cruise ships and causes diarrhoea and vomiting

Symptoms vary in different individuals. Common symptoms include:

- Persistent sensation of bobbing, rocking, swinging, swaying, floating or tumbling
- Tiredness
- Headache and nausea
- Difficulty concentrating
- Loss of self-confidence

Symptoms are usually relieved when in motion, e.g., riding in a car. MDS does not include the usual symptoms of vestibular (inner ear) problems, such as a spinning sensation, pain, tinnitus, deafness, or double vision. Unfortunately, MDS may persist for months or even years.

DIAGNOSIS & TREATMENT

The diagnosis is usually clinical, made by a combination of the patient's history, examination and the exclusion of reasonable alternatives. There is usually a history of a sea journey or other motion, then a return to a normal environment, followed by the start of the symptoms. Symptoms start immediately within days of travel and not in weeks or months.

MDS is a self-limiting condition. Some people are helped with a vestibular training programme, particularly if they also have balance problems due to an inner ear dysfunction. If this training programme is started one week before travel, these exercises will raise your tolerance and may help in preventing this condition.

ADVICE FOR HEALTH-CARE PROFESSIONALS

1. The usual anti-sickness medications do not help.
2. Benzodiazepines have been shown to the most benefit for both prevention and treatment. For prevention, a small dose should be given six hours before travel and then every eight hours during the journey.
3. Balance rehabilitation physical therapy has a small benefit.
4. Anti-depressants help some to cope with the symptoms.

ADVICE FOR PATIENTS & CARERS

Although there is no single, established method of symptom management, some useful coping tips include:

1. Reducing stress, as stress has been known to be a trigger for severity of symptoms.
2. Getting a good night's sleep is vital, as tiredness can exacerbate symptoms.
3. Symptoms can be improved by pressing an acupressure point called "pericardium 6", which is located on the inside of the forearm, above two inches about the crease of the wrist. Pressing on this point using the index finger of the opposite hand or wearing a wristband can be helpful.
4. Ginger has been reported to improve symptoms.
5. Join a support group. This will help you to recognize that there are many people in the world who suffer from this condition.
6. Regular gentle exercise, like yoga or tai chi, helps to relieve stress and improve balance.
7. Rocking chair during sedentary activity as symptoms improve with movements

SUMMARY

MDS is an uncommon but frustrating disease. It is not a serious condition, but it is life-changing. Most people live a normal life, but it will require a positive mental attitude, lifestyle changes, and possibly some medication. More research is needed into this condition.

FURTHER READING

1. Gordon CR, Spitzer O, Shupak A, Doweckl. "Survey of Mal de Debarquement". BMJ. 1992; 304:544.
2. Cohen, H. "Vertigo after sailing a nineteenth century ship". Journal of Vestibular Research. 1996; 6:31-5.
3. Brown JJ, Baloh, RW. "Persistent Mal de Debarquement syndrome: a motion-induced subjective disorder of balance". American Journal of Otolaryngology 1987; 8:19.
4. Hain, TC, Hanna, PA, Rheinberger, MA. "Mal De Debarquement". Arch Otolaryngol Head Neck Surg 1999; 125: 615-620.
5. Murphy, TP. "Mal De Debarquement syndrome: a forgotten entity?" Otolaryngology Head & Neck Surgery1993; 109: 10-3.
6. Zimbelman, JL, Walton, TM. "Vestibular rehabilitation of a patient with persistant Mal De Debarquement". Physical Therapy Case Report 1992:2(4):129-137.
7. Grontved, A, Brask, T, Kambskard, J, Hentzer, E. "Ginger root against seasickness.A controlled trial on the open sea". Acta Otolaryngol.105.1-2 (1998): 45-49.

Chapter 9

Dizziness in multiple sclerosis (MS)

Case study: A fifty-year-old who had been previously diagnosed with MS was referred to a neurology clinic with a history of dizziness associated with rotational vertigo, difficulty in mobilizing and disturbed sleep, which had been evident for the last 6 months. Her GP prescribed various medications, in addition to a range of homeopathic and herbal medications that she bought herself, but they did not provide any relief. Her dizziness and vertigo symptoms were making her anxious and she started to have panic attacks. In the hospital clinic, she was thoroughly examined and special scans including MRI (magnetic resonance imaging) were undertaken, but all returned normal results. She was then referred for vestibular rehabilitation therapy. After a detailed assessment by a physical therapist, she was started on a programme of vestibular rehabilitation exercises and within three months, her symptoms improved significantly and she was able to mobilise and sleep better.

INTRODUCTION

Multiple sclerosis is a degenerative disease of the brain and spinal cord. This condition typically affects the eyes (loss of vision) and patients also report weakness in the legs. Vertigo is present in about 10% of MS suffers.

CAUSES & SYMPTOMS

The exact cause of vertigo in MS patients is not fully understood, however dizziness can result when the disease start involving the balance organs such as cerebellum, brainstem. Anxiety and depression which may be present up to 25% of MS suffers can contribute to the symptoms of dizziness and vertigo. Problems in the inner ear may also cause balance disturbance.

Dizziness may present with a spinning sensation, where the surroundings appear to rotate, or a rushing sensation where the ground appears to suddenly rush forward. Vertigo is unlikely to persist for a long time in MS patients, although improvements are slow. However, it may leave a chronic vertigo sensation and susceptibility to motion sickness.

DIAGNOSIS & TREATMENT

The diagnosis of dizziness in MS patient is usually made after taking a detailed history, performing thorough examination and with out investigations. However, occasionally investigations are required, such as an MRI scan of the brain, to look for further worsening of the disease.

Drug treatment

1. Anti-motion sickness (antiemetic) such as Prochlorperazine is quite commonly used. Hyosine is also used both as tablets and as a skin patch.
2. In severe cases, a short case of corticosteroids is used to improve symptoms.
3. Benzodiazepine e.g. diazepam is used if severe anxiety is an associated feature.
4. Betahistine is used to reduce the pressure in the inner ear by improving the circulation. This in turn may improve the symptoms. This can take up to three months to produce a good effect.
5. Complementary treatments like Gingko Biloba and ginger capsules or ginger tea are claimed to increase blood flow and improve vertigo and nausea.

Exercise treatment

1. Repositioning manoeuvre like Epley's or the Brandt Daroff manoeuvre can be performed at home or in the hospital clinic.
2. Acupuncture and cranial osteopathy are reported to be effective in some patients.

3. Vestibular rehabilitation therapy (VRT) is extremely effective. This will help to retrain the brain to recognize and process signals from the inner ear (vestibular system) and co-ordinate the information from eyes, muscles and joints. This commonly includes desensitising the balance system to the movements that provoke vertigo. VRT is usually very successful in alleviating the problem.
4. Tai chi has been proven to benefit MS sufferers balance problems

ADVICE FOR HEALTH-CARE PROFESSIONALS

1. Side effects of anti-emetics include tiredness, drowsiness, muscular and joint stiffness. Some patients may develop features of Parkinson's disease, such as muscle stiffness and tremors, which disappear with the cessation of medication.
2. Early referral for VRT may provide a long-term solution to the problem

ADVICE FOR PATIENTS & CARERS

1. It is worth explaining to your relatives or carer that vertigo symptoms may be worse when lying down. If you are lying down, try to use two pillows and monitor the sufferer until the symptoms subside.
2. The symptoms are usually worst first thing in the morning and they generally improve as the day progresses, so take extra care in the early morning.
3. Keeping dim lights on at night will help you to walk. Using a walking stick or using walls or a lamppost for guidance can help with navigation.
4. Walking barefoot can also help with moving about in the house, although there is a possibility of injury to the toes.
5. Keep a diary of your symptoms and take it with you to your doctor.

SUMMARY

Dizziness with or without spinning sensation is a common symptom among MS patients. Accurate diagnosis is important in getting the best treatment. Medications can provide some relief. VRT may provide effective and long-term relief.

FURTHER READING

1. Freeman JA, Langdon DW, Hobart JC, Thompson AJ. The impact of inpatient rehabilitation on progressive multiple sclerosis. *Annals of Neurology* 1997; 42:236–44.
2. Solari A, Filippini G, Gasco P *et al.* Physical rehabilitation has a positive effect on disability in multiple sclerosis patients. *Neurology* 1999; 52:57–62.
3. Patti F, Ciancio MR, Reggio E *et al.* The impact of outpatient rehabilitation quality of life in multiple sclerosis. *Journal of Neurology* 2002; 249:1027–33.
4. Jones L, Lewis Y, Harrison J *et al.* The effectiveness of occupational therapy and physiotherapy in multiple sclerosis patients with ataxia of the upper limb and trunk. *Clinical Rehabilitation* 1996; 10: 277–82.
5. Armutlu K, Karabudak R, Nurlu G. Physiotherapy approaches in the treatment of ataxic multiple sclerosis: a pilot study. *Neurorehabilitation & Neural Repair* 2001; 15: 203–11.

Chapter 10

Dizziness in Parkinson's disease

Case history. A 65-year-old Parkinson's sufferer was seen in a neurology clinic with a frequent history of dizziness and falls, particularly after getting up from sitting position. A thorough examination did not reveal any abnormalities. His anti-Parkinson's medications were reduced and at two months' follow-up, he reported some improvement in his symptoms. Although his dizziness symptoms did not disappear completely, he was able to manage better.

INTRODUCTION

Parkinson's disease is a very common neurodegenerative disorder that is characterised by a progressive loss of muscle control, leading to tremors at rest, slowness, and disorders of balance. As the disease progresses, it becomes difficult for the patient to walk, talk and complete simple tasks. Dizziness is not only unpleasant, but also dangerous, as it may lead to falls and broken bones. Dizziness is not part of the diagnostic criteria for Parkinson's disease – however, all of the symptoms of Parkinson's disease, such as tremors, stiffness, and difficulty walking, may lead to dizziness.

CAUSES & SYMPTOMS

- Postural hypotension. This condition is characterised by a fall in blood pressure on standing from a lying or sitting position. Normally when we stand up from a lying or sitting position, the blood pools in the legs and our muscles and blood vessels work to squeeze the blood back to the heart. A compensatory increase in heart rate maintains blood pressure. If this process of pumping blood back to the heart does not work, it will lead to postural hypotension, which may cause dizziness. Postural hypotension increases as the disease progresses, and dehydration can exacerbate the problem.

- Medication side effect. The medication used to treat Parkinson's disease, such as Sinemet, can cause dizziness. Those taking tablets for blood pressure may have a compounding effect.
- The loss of balance can be caused by the lack of fine control of the muscles that accompanies Parkinson's disease. This may lead to a loss of confidence and strength, but can also be improved by physical therapy.
- Other causes. It is possible that people with Parkinson's disease are also suffering from other conditions causing dizziness not directly related to the disease itself (e.g. benign paroxysmal positional vertigo, labyrinthitis).

DIAGNOSIS & TREATMENT

The diagnosis of dizziness in Parkinson's disease is usually made with detailed history and examination. Occasionally, a special scan, such as an MRI, is needed. Treatment is described below.

ADVICE FOR HEALTH-CARE PROFESSIONALS

1. Nausea is less common with modified release Sinemet, which is more slowly absorbed than the regular Sinemet. Nausea can also be prevented by slowly increasing the dose. If required, Domperidone (Motilium) can be given for the prevention and treatment of nausea.
2. Dizziness due to postural hypotension may improve with time.
3. When low blood pressure is a side effect of medication, this can be treated by reducing the dose or changing to other medications.

ADVICE FOR PATIENTS & CARERS

1. In some Parkinson's sufferers, low blood pressure can lead to dizziness, particularly in the first few days of treatment, and so care should be taken when driving or operating machinery.

2. To help prevent dizziness due to low blood pressure, it is important to keep hydrated. The colour of urine can indicate the level of dehydration. The colour should be light yellow – if it is dark like apple juice, then you are dehydrated.

3. Heavy meals can cause low blood pressure by moving lots of blood to the stomach, so small and more frequent meals may help. Avoid excess alcohol, as this may lead to dehydration due to a diuretic effect.

4. A physiotherapist and/or rehabilitation therapist may help to improve dizziness.

5. Maintaining increased salt intake (about 10g per day) may reduce the incidence of hypotension.

6. Standing up slowly may give more time to the blood vessels in the legs to constrict. This can avoid collapse.

SUMMARY

Dizziness in Parkinson's disease can be caused by a variety of reasons. Most causes can be identified and treated effectively. This may require an assessment by a neurologist and physical therapist. Most patient can improve their symptoms of dizziness by either alteration in their medications or physical exercise.

FURTHER READING

1. www.parkinsons.org.uk
2. www.patient.co.uk

Chapter 11

Fibromyalgia and dizziness

Case study: A 38-year-old piano teacher and church musician had a long history of recurrent "colds" and viral infections. Despite not having a particularly stressful or busy life, he frequently had sleep disturbances, tiredness, aches and pains, depression and feelings of dizziness. After visiting various specialists, including a GP, neurologist, rheumatologist, orthopaedics and ear, nose and throat surgeons, he was finally diagnosed with fibromyalgia. His therapy, including pills, exercise, counseling, and finally leaving his job, improved the clinical condition.

INTRODUCTION

Fibromyalgia is a rare illness characterised by sleep disturbance, chronic fatigue, and widespread musculoskeletal pains. Whilst the cause is still unknown, there is some evidence to suggest that genetic factors may play a role in the development of fibromyalgia, as there is a high aggregation of fibromyalgia within families. Some researchers believe this is due to psychiatric disorder, while others attribute it to a chronic viral illness.

CAUSES & SYMPTOMS

The most likely cause for dizziness in fibromyalgia is the body's inability to regulate blood pressure, which significantly falls upon standing up from a sitting or lying position. This leads to dizziness, sweating, weakness, and lightheadedness, and in certain situations, people may fall. This is called neural mediated hypotension.

In normal circumstances, when a person stands up, the blood rushes to their feet and legs, which reduces the amount of blood returning to the heart. The body releases adrenaline, which causes blood vessels in the legs to constrict. This increases the flow of blood to the heart and also increases the heart rate. This effect causes the heart to pump more blood to the rest of the body to compensate for blood that went to the legs.

In neurally mediated hypotension, this process does not work due to a failure of the interaction between the heart and the brain, despite both being structurally normal. When these patients get up from a sitting or lying position, there is no constriction of the blood vessels and the heart rate does not increase, so the blood pressure falls. This leads to the above symptoms.

DIAGNOSIS & TREATMENT

A diagnosis of dizziness in fibromyalgia sufferers is usually made by performing a tilt table test. The patient is strapped on a table with various equipment attached for monitoring blood pressure and heart rate. Observations are taken twice: once whilst the patient is lying flat, and once immediately after the table is put into the upright position. Changes in perceived dizziness and physiological measures are compared between body positions.

Treatment involves a combination of increased salt and water intake, in conjunction with drugs that regulate blood pressure. The treatment is not curative, but helps to control the symptoms. There is no single treatment available for fibromyalgia. However, treatment commonly involves the use of antidepressants, acupuncture, painkillers, and exercises.

ADVICE FOR HEALTH-CARE PROFESSIONALS

1. Head-up tilt table testing can be used to evaluate autonomic dysfunction (neural mediated hypotension) and is frequently helpful for the work-up of fibromyalgia (FM) complaints, including fatigue, dizziness, and palpitations.
2. Dizziness, syncope or fainting is likely to occur in susceptible patients during tilt table testing.
3. The tilt test can also provoke seizure. It is important to keep emergency medications where the tilt test is done.

4. Other causes of dizziness, such as benign paroxysmal positional vertigo, labyrinthitis, and Meniere's disease can also cause symptoms in fibromyalgia patients and would need appropriate treatment.

ADVICE FOR PATIENTS & CARERS

1. The test may take up to 90 minutes to complete. The results are usually available the same day.
2. If the test is positive, there is effective treatment available which will alleviate the dizziness symptoms significantly.

SUMMARY

Dizziness in fibromyalgia may be caused by neural mediated hypotension. This dizziness can be quite disabling in fibromyalgia suffers. It can be reliably diagnosed with a tilt table test. The symptoms of dizziness can be improved with various medications.

FURTHER READING

1. National Fibromyalgia Association (www.fmaware.org)
2. http://www.fibromyalgia-symptoms.org/fibromyalgia_dizziness.html
3. http://www.fibromyalgiasyndrome.co.uk/balance-problems-dizziness.html

Chapter 12

Dizziness in children

Case Study: A 20-month-old boy was presented to the doctor as suffering from gait abnormality (falling to the left side while walking) and vomiting. His father reported that these symptoms had lasted for about a day, and told paramedics that his child was falling more frequently. He was referred to the paediatric emergency assessment unit, where a scan of the brain (CT, computerised tomogram) and lumbar puncture (fluid taken from the spine) were undertaken. All tests came back as normal, and so the boy was admitted for 24 hours for observation in the children's ward. There was no improvement in this time period, and he was referred to a tertiary paediatric centre, where another brain scan (MRI) was done. He was subsequently diagnosed with cerebellum infarction (a type of stroke). No specific treatment was given. He was referred for stroke rehabilitation and within a few months, he made an excellent recovery.

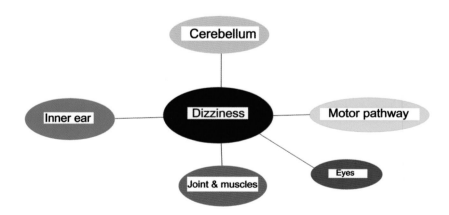

Causes of dizziness in children

Fig 12.0

INTRODUCTION

Dizziness in children is a vague diagnosis that can describe various conditions, including lightheadedness, anxiety, intoxication, visual problems, weakness, depression and vertigo. It is not easy to diagnose dizziness in children. This may be due to the inability of some children to describe their symptoms, which makes their evaluation difficult. However, a detailed review of their history and a thorough physical examination can establish a diagnosis in most cases.

CAUSES & SYMPTOMS

Common (less serious) conditions causing dizziness:

- Benign paroxysmal positional vertigo of childhood
- Labyrinthitis
- Migraine
- Motion sickness
- Otitis media
- Anaemia
- Anxiety and Depression
- Hyperventilation, orthostatic hypotension, and presyncope
- Inner ear problems (cholesteatoma, meniers disease, mastoiditis, and perilymph fistula)
- Epilepsy (seizure)
- Visual (eye) abnormalities

More serious conditions causing dizziness:

- Infection of the central nervous system
- Trauma to the head and/or ear
- Stroke
- Poisoning or the side effects of medication
- Arrhythmias (irregular heartbeat)
- Tumour

Children present with a variety of symptoms, as outlined above. However, the following would suggest dizziness caused by inner ear dysfunction:

1. Deafness and tinnitus
2. Motion sensitivity
3. Clumsiness
4. Recurrent falls
5. Nystagmus and vomiting
6. Balance problems in the dark
7. Behavior abnormalities
8. Developmental and reflex delays. The child may have decreased development of eye-hand and eye-foot co-ordination: hopping, riding a bicycle, stair climbing with alternating legs, etc.

Children can have similar vestibular dysfunctions as adults. Benign paroxysmal positional vertigo is usually present after trauma. It may also begin after cochlear implant surgery or vestibular labyrinthitis. Migrainous vertigo may present with vertigo without headaches.

Children also have two specific disorders related to vestibular dysfunction:

1. **Benign paroxysmal positional vertigo of childhood** is a disorder usually seen in children of 2-12 years of age. During the attack, the children appears frightened and off balance, often trying to reach for something to hold. This may be associated with sweating, nystagmus, nausea and vomiting. These brief episodes usually recur many times a day for several days and are then followed by symptom free periods before recurring again. There is usually a family history of migraine. The examination is usually normal in between episodes. Some children may subsequently develop migraine.
2. **Paroxysmal torticollis of infancy** is a self-limiting condition consists of recurrent episodes of head tilt followed by vomiting,

pallor, agitation and ataxia. The individual attack lasts for hours, and occasionally for days. This condition gets better gradually and usually disappears before the age of 5. It is considered as a variant of migraine in children.

DIAGNOSIS & TREATMENT

Collecting a detailed history of the child that covers all of the above causes is extremely important, and preferably should be undertaken in the presence of a parent or a carer. A thorough physical examination with particular attention to neurological and vestibular functions should be performed. Various investigations may be needed to establish the diagnosis, including blood tests, brain scan, and lumbar puncture (fluid from the spine, after excluding increased intracranial pressure).

Vestibular rehabilitation therapy is extremely effective for children. Typically, children respond better than adults, due to their ability to compensate quickly. Furthermore, children are less fearful and tend to participate well in balance rehabilitation. Vestibular rehabilitation therapy is effective in eliminating vertigo symptoms, improving motor development, improving balance and co-ordination, and promoting normal growth in children with dizziness.

ADVICE FOR HEALTH-CARE PROFESSIONALS

1. Dizziness, abnormal gait, headaches and vomiting can be a sign of a stroke.
2. A significant whiplash-type injury can damage an artery (the basilar artery) that supplies blood to the balance organs, leading to dizziness.
3. Most children will have otitis media, BPPV, or migraine as the cause of their dizziness. However, if there is head trauma, decreased conscious level, or meningitis, an urgent brain scan is needed.
4. Most children do respond very well to vestibular rehabilitation.

ADVICE FOR PATIENTS & CARERS

1. Keep a diary of the dizzy spells and associated symptoms.
2. Reassure and calm the child, as the underlying cause could be anxiety.
3. Most causes of dizziness in children are not serious.
4. Make sure that the child is well hydrated and eat a balanced diet.
5. You must consult the doctor if the child develops any signs or symptoms of serious illness or if you have any particular concerns.

SUMMARY

Dizziness in children is a common problem, and it is not easy to diagnose and treat, as children may describe dizziness in different ways. Symptoms include light-headedness, anxiety, ataxia (balance problems), hyperventilation, visual disturbance, and true vertigo. However, a careful and detailed history and examination will establish the diagnosis in most cases. Vestibular rehabilitation therapy is usually very successful.

FURTHER READING

1. Bower, CM, Cotton, RT. "The spectrum of vertigo in children". Arch Otolaryngol Head Neck Surg 1995; 121:911.
2. Ravid, S, Bienkowski, R, Eviater, L. "A simplified diagnostic approach to dizziness in children". Padiatr Neurol 2003:29:317.
3. Riina, N, llmari, P, Kentala, E. "Vertigo and imbalance in children: a retrospective study in a Helsinki University otorhinolaryngology clinic". Arch Otolaryngol Head Neck Surg 2005; 131:1996.
4. Casselbrant, ML, Mandel, EM. "Balance disorders in children". Neurol Clin 2005; 23:807
5. Tusa, RJ, Saada AA, Jr, Niparko, JK. "Dizziness in childhood". J Child Neurol 1994; 9:261

Chapter 13

Dizziness after injury

Case study: A 25-year-old rally driver was involved in an accident in which his car rolled over several times. He developed intense dizziness, deafness in the left ear, and weakness on the left side of his face. He was admitted to the hospital where a scan of the head and neck confirmed a fracture of the skull bone (temporal bone). He was treated in a propped-up position and was given medications for nausea and vomiting. He was discharged one week later. His hearing never returned to normal. His facial weakness and dizziness improved with the treatment offered by the physiotherapist.

INTRODUCTION

Dizziness is a frequent symptom in people who suffer an injury to the head and/or neck region. The injuries following road traffic accidents, assaults, falls and contact sports such as rugby, football, and kickboxing can cause dizziness (including vertigo). The likely reason for developing vertigo after trauma is the release of otoconia (calcium crystals) from the utricle to the semicircular canals (in the inner ear). The symptoms and treatment are dependent upon the severity of the injury and underlying structure involved. It is extremely important to get appropriate diagnosis from a medical professional, and this can often lead to successful treatment.

CAUSES & SYMPTOMS

The following are common causes of injury-related dizziness:

1. **Benign paroxysmal positional vertigo (BPPV).** This is the most common type of vertigo induced by injury. The vertigo is produced when the head is placed in certain positions. It is

usually treated with Epley's manoeuvre. Over 95% of people get better with this treatment.

2. **Meniere's disease.** One possible underlying cause is bleeding in the inner ear. This may lead to disturbance of fluid transport and increase pressure, leading to the symptoms of Menier's disease such as deafness, tinnitus and vertigo. These symptoms could start immediately, or may appear up to 12 months after the accident.

3. **Migraine.** There is a high incidence of migraine after a head injury. It is important to exclude other causes of dizziness and headache following head injury, such as bleeding in the brain and fracture of the skull bones. The treatment includes painkillers, anti-sickness medications and rehabilitation in some patients.

4. **Perilymph fistula.** Perilymph fistula is an abnormal communication between the middle and the internal ear. This can happen following an injury. Symptoms of dizziness and imbalance start after straining or blowing the nose. There is also the possibility of dizziness following a loud noise (Tullio's phenomenon). Operative repair is sometimes needed with this condition.

5. **Psychogenic vertigo** Psychogenic vertigo may develop following the injury. The symptoms are more common in younger female patients. Sufferers report long-lasting dizziness, nausea, headaches, breathlessness, anxiety and palpitations. The symptoms may be aggravated by a stressful situation. Typically, examinations return no obvious cause of this condition, and patients are referred for psychiatric treatment.

6. **Post-concussion syndrome** Post-concussion syndrome is a complex disorder in which headaches and dizziness can last for months following head injury. The other symptoms include anxiety, irritability, tiredness – which may affect sleep pattern – and a loss of concentration and memory. There is usually a history of loss of consciousness following a head injury. The symptoms usually start within one week of the accident and disappear in about 12 weeks. There is no specific treatment available. However, some patients may require medication for nausea and vomiting.

7. **Whiplash injury syndrome (WIS)** WIS is similar to post-concussion syndrome, with additional symptoms of pain in the neck and upper back muscles. The symptoms usually last longer than six months. Occasionally a special scan (magnetic resonance scan) of the neck may be required to exclude any injury to the spine. The severity of symptoms is dependent on speed of impact. Treatments consist of painkillers, muscle relaxants, physiotherapy, and some people benefit from chiropractic treatment.

DIAGNOSIS & TREATMENT

The diagnosis is usually made by taking detailed history of trauma and examination while considering the above causes. Treatment is individualised to the diagnosis. Treatment usually includes a combination of medication, changes in life style, and possibly physical therapy. Occasionally, surgery may be required.

ADVICE FOR HEALTH-CARE PROFESSIONALS:

1. Treatment failures are very likely due to misdiagnosis.
2. Follow up is extremely important to review the original diagnosis and to check progress.
3. There is a high litigation rate in cases of dizziness secondary to injury.

ADVICE FOR PATIENTS & CARES

1. Post-injury dizziness can be treated at home with exercises.
2. If the symptoms are very severe or do not improve in three weeks of home exercises, then seek medical advice.
3. In most cases of dizziness following injury, the underlying cause is not serious.

SUMMARY

Dizziness after trauma is quite common. Special tests may be required to exclude injury to the brain and surrounding structures.

In the majority of patients, these vertigo symptoms improve with time. However, early treatment will expedite the recovery. Occasionally, surgical treatment is needed.

FURTHER READING

1. Ernst A, Basta D, Seidl RO, Todt L, Schere H, Clarke A. "Management of posttraumatic vertigo". Otolaryngol Head Neck Surg. 2005 Apr; 132(4): 554-8
2. Feneley, M. R. and P. Murthy (1994). "Acute bilateral vestibulo-cochlear dysfunction following occipital fracture". J Laryngol Otol 108(1): 54-6
3. Rubin, AM. "Dizziness associated with head-neck trauma". Audio Digest Vol 30 #22, 1997
4. Hoffer, ME et al. "Characterising and treating dizziness after mild head trauma". Oto Neurol 25:135-138,2004

Chapter 14

Dizziness in old age

Case study: A 85-year-old lady was brought by her daughter to the Dizzyclear clinic complaining of intense dizziness with spinning sensations when she lay in her bed at night. She also experienced the same symptoms on getting out of bed. She was otherwise in good health. The examination confirmed that she was suffering from benign paroxysmal positional vertigo. Modified Epley's manoeuvre completely resolved her symptoms within four days of treatment.

INTRODUCTION

Dizziness is extremely common in patients over 60. It is estimated that up to 30% of patients over 60 suffer from dizziness. Dizziness can have a detrimental effect on quality of life. Dizziness can also lead to anxiety and depression. Dizziness is also a common reason for elderly patients to fall.

CAUSES & SYMPTOMS:

The common causes include the following:
- Peripheral (inner-ear) related. This is the commonest cause for patients to develop dizziness. Benign paroxysmal positional vertigo (BPPV) is the leading reason. This can be safely treated at home with the Epley's manoeuvre. Other less common causes of dizziness include labyrinthitis and Meniere's disease.
- Central (brainstem and cerebellar) cause. This group includes dizziness secondary to stroke. The symptoms include imbalance, lack of co-coordination and speech, nausea, and illusion of motion (appearance of movement in a static image) that may last for years following a stroke.
- Proprioception (damage to the nerves in the feet). Loss of sensation in the feet, which may be due to diabetes. Vitamin B12 deficiency is another cause of dizziness.

- Medication side effects. Elderly patients are on a lot of medications for various conditions and the side effects of many of them may cause dizziness. The following conditions and medication are known to cause dizziness:

1) Anti-epilepsy medications such as phenytoin and carbmazepine
2) Blood pressure medications such as propanolol, Isosorbide, Furosemide, Nifedipine
3) Anti-sickness medications such as meclizine, scopolamine, Promethazine
4) Tricyclic antidepressants such as Nortriptyline
5) Anti-Parkinson's medication such as Sinemet
6) Medications for heartburn such as Cimetidine, Lansoprazole
7) Other drugs such as benzodiazepines, gentamicin, Cis-platinum, Phenothiazines

- Other causes. Other less common causes include anxiety, depression, eye (visual) problems and cervical spondylosis (arthritis of the neck). Abnormal heart rhythm can cause dizziness, but this is usually associated with fainting episodes. It is possible that in about quarter of these patients, no obvious cause may be found.

DIAGNOSIS & TREATMENT

The diagnosis is usually made by taking history and conducting an examination, without investigations. However, the following tests may be useful:

1. Scan of the brain to confirm or exclude stroke
2. Blood tests may help to exclude vitamin B12 deficiency anemia

Treatment depends upon the underlying cause. However, the following treatments are usually recommended:

1. Epley's manoeuvre for the treatment of vertigo (BPPV). If the diagnosis is confirmed, a modified home Epley's manoeuvre can be safely done (see chapter 23).

2. Chronic dizziness will benefit from vestibular rehabilitation therapy (see chapter 22).
3. Walking aids may be needed to prevent falls secondary to dizziness.

ADVICE FOR HEALTH-CARE PROFESSIONALS:

1. Dizziness is unlikely to be caused by a stroke: common causes should be considered first.
2. Investigations are rarely helpful in the diagnosis of dizziness in older patients.
3. Anxiety and poor vision often accompany dizziness, but are rarely the only cause.

ADVICE FOR PATIENTS & CARERS:

Dizziness is extremely common in the elderly population, so get help early from your GP. Do not suffer in silence.

1. Keep a diary of your symptoms.
2. Take a friend with you to see the doctor.
3. Most causes can be treated safely at home or in the GP's surgery.

SUMMARY

Dizziness in the elderly has numerous causes and should be regarded as a significant symptom. All elderly patients should be screened for symptoms of dizziness including depression and anxiety. Good assessment and treatment for this common condition can significantly improve the symptoms.

FURTHER READING

1. Grimby, A, Rosenhall, U. "Health-related quality of life and dizziness in old age". Gerontology, 1995:41(5): 286-98.
2. Uneri, A, Polat, S. "Vertigo, dizziness and imbalance in the elderly". J Laryngol Otol 2008; 122(5) 466-9.

3. Tinetti, ME, Williams, CS, Gill TM. "Dizziness among older adults: a possible geriatric syndrome". Ann Intern Med. 2000:132:337-344.
4. Colledge, NR, Barr-Hamilton, RM, Lewis, SJ, Sellar, RK, Wilson, JA. "Evaluation of investigations to diagnose the cause of dizziness in elderly people: a community-based controlled study". BMJ. 1996:313:788-792.
5. Oghalai, JS, Manolidis, S, Barth, JL, Stewart, MG, Jenkins, HA. "Unrecognised benign positional vertigo in elderly patients". Otolaryngol Head Neck Surg. 2000:122:630-634.

Chapter 15

Microvascular compression (MVC)

Case study. A fifty-two-year old attended a neurology clinic, having suffered from brief attacks of vertigo, tinnitus, nausea, motion intolerance and deafness over the previous year. These attacks used to last for a few hours, after which most symptoms would improve. After an MRI scan, he was diagnosed with MVC of the eighth nerve, which is concerned with hearing and balance. He was prescribed medication (carbmazepine), which improved his symptoms. About eighteen months after the treatment, the symptoms became worse again. The patient was referred to a neurosurgeon in the United States for microvascular decompression (MVD) and made a complete recovery.

CAUSES & SYMPTOMS

MVC syndrome is a group of conditions where symptoms are caused by compression of the cranial nerves by blood vessels, causing the symptoms. Surgical treatment to relieve the symptoms is called microvascular decompression. There are three well-known conditions:

1. Symptoms due to compression of the fifth cranial nerve include facial pains on one side of the face. This nerve is called the trigeminal nerve and provides sensation to the skin of the face. This condition is called "trigeminal neuralgia" or "Tic Doloroux". The patient typically complains of severe pain on one side of the face that may be exacerbated by touch or irritation of the face. This condition is well-recognised and numerous cases have reported success after MVD.
2. Symptoms caused by compression of the seventh cranial nerve include short episodes of spasm of the facial muscles – known as hemi-facial spasms – since this nerve supplies the muscles of

the face. There have been many reports of successful treatment with the surgical treatment (MVD).

3. Symptoms due to compression of the eighth cranial nerve include repeated short episodes of vertigo, deafness, tinnitus, and nausea. This nerve is concerned with hearing and balance function. This is not a common condition and a limited number of cases have been diagnosed and improved with the treatment.

DIAGNOSIS & TREATMENT

There is no single diagnostic test available for MVC. However, a magnetic resonance imaging (MRI) scan is the most likely test to identify the blood vessel compressing the nerve. In addition, a hearing test may show deafness.

Medical treatment

The medications that provide relief of symptoms include carbmazepine and phenytoin, typically used to treat epilepsy. If there is partial response, then another medication called Baclofen may be added.

Surgical treatment

Repositioning of the blood vessel covering the nerve with keyhole surgery is a well-known treatment for this condition and can be performed with minimal complications. This procedure is called microvascular decompression (MVD), and most patients are able to go home on the same day. This treatment was pioneered in 1984 by Dr. Peter Jannetta, a neurosurgeon from Pittsburgh.

FURTHER RESEARCH

At present, further research is being undertaken to explore new methods of diagnosing and managing this condition. So far, only a limited number of cases been treated surgically worldwide.

ADVICE FOR HEALTH-CARE PROFESSIONALS:

1. MVC is a rare cause of vertigo and should be considered if other causes for vertigo, deafness, or tinnitus are not present. This may be an incidental finding following a brain scan.
2. Medications may take a few months to have full effect.
3. Surgical treatment is still in the early stages of its development.

ADVICE FOR PATIENTS & CARERS:

1. There is limited information available over the internet about this condition. However, the following website provides some reliable information: http://www.american-hearing.org/disor ders/microvascular-compression-syndrome
2. The underlying cause is usually not serious.

SUMMARY

MVC is a rare cause of vertigo, deafness, tinnitus and balance problems. This condition is caused by a blood vessel compressing the vestibulocochlear nerve, which is concerned with both hearing and balance. It is usually diagnosed with an MRI scan. A few cases have been successfully treated by medications and surgery (MVD).

FURTHER READING:

1. Applebaum EL, Valvasori, GE. "Auditory and vestibular system findings in patients with vascular loops in the internal audtitory canal". Ann ORL 92(112): 63-69, 1984
2. Brackmann, DE, Kesser BW, Day, JD. "Microvascular decompression of the vestibulocochlear nerve for disabling positional vertigo: the house ear clinic experience". Oto Neurotol 22:882-887, 2001

3. Janetta, PJ, Moller, MB, Moller, AR. "Disabling positional vertigo". NEJM 310:1700-1705, 1984
4. McCabe, BF, Harker, LA. "Vascular loop as a cause of vertigo". Ann ORL 92:542-543, 1983
5. Moller, MB. "Vascular compression of the eighth cranial nerve as a cause of vertigo". Keio J. Med 40(3) 146-150, 1991

Chapter 16

Psychogenic dizziness

Case study: A forty-two-year old was referred to the Dizzyclear clinic with a twelve-month history of dizziness following a road traffic accident in which she was the driver of a car that collided with an oncoming motor cyclist at high speed. The motorcyclist was killed. Her GP tried various medications for dizziness, with no success. Previously, she experienced dizzy episodes at night, which had woken her from sleep numerous times. A full ear, nose and throat examination was performed, in addition to a brain scan, but all returned normal. She was referred to a psychiatrist and was diagnosed with post-traumatic stress disorder. She was offered treatment in the form of medication and psychotherapy. Within three months of treatment, she reported improvement in her dizziness symptoms.

INTRODUCTION

Psychogenic dizziness is a condition characterised by a recurring or continuous problem with balance. The patient may not have the classical symptoms of spinning dizziness caused by inner ear problems, but instead have chronic subjective dizziness, which produces a feeling of swaying, often triggered by crowds of people, flashing lights, heavy traffic or any stressful situation. Most tests for diagnosing inner ear problems, such as a hearing test and brain scan, are usually normal. About 15% of chronically dizzy patients have psychogenic dizziness. It is more common in younger patients who have a history of anxiety, panic attacks characterised by headaches, breathlessness, palpitations, nausea, and sleep disturbance. Treatment is usually offered by a psychiatrist.

Psychogenic dizziness is usually a diagnosis of exclusion. Various underlying psychiatric conditions can cause dizziness. However, chronic dizziness can also lead to various psychiatric conditions. The diagnosis of psychogenic dizziness should be discussed with the patient just like any other illness. When it is explained how the mechanisms of thoughts and emotions may induce somatic symptoms, most people will recognise and understand their condition. Once the psychological issues are addressed with empathy, symptoms may resolve completely.

CAUSES & SYMPTOMS

The following psychological conditions either cause dizziness or result from chronic dizziness:

1. **Panic and anxiety attacks**. These are not easy to diagnose, and are either the result of dizziness or can cause dizziness. Patients usually complain of symptoms of anxiety such as a lump in the throat, chest pain, shortness of breath without obvious cause, difficulty in going to sleep and other vague symptoms that are difficult to diagnose.
2. **Depression**. Dizziness due to depression is usually described as a "swimming sensation" or inability to concentrate. Patients may also have other symptoms of depression, such as low mood, tiredness, early morning awakening, lack of appetite, or hopelessness. Most antidepressants can impair balance to some extent. However, an appropriate dose is necessary to provide relief with fewer side effects.
3. **Phobic postural vertigo**. Most patients complain of spontaneous postural vertigo and unsteadiness in maintaining an upright posture and walking. Sometimes this is induced by a stimulus such as a visit to a shopping centre or going in a lift. The diagnosis usually involve the following six criteria: (1) dizziness and subjective disturbance of balance while standing or walking, despite normal balance tests (2) fluctuating unsteadiness for seconds to minutes or momentary perception of illusory body perturbations (3) usually a perceptual stimuli or social situation as a provoking factor with a tendency for rapid conditioning, generalisation, and

avoidance behaviour (4) anxiety and vegetative symptoms during or after vertigo (5) obsessive-compulsive personality type, labile effect or mild depression and (6) onset frequently after a period of emotional stress, serious illness, or a vestibular disorder. These patients are usually treated by psychotherapy (including autogenic training AT) and cognitive behaviour therapy.

4. **Acrophobia and agoraphobia.** Acrophobia is a condition where a person develops a fear of heights. People suffering from acrophobia can have panic attacks while looking down from a height. Agoraphobia refers to a fear of open spaces. People suffering from agoraphobia dread being in or crossing open places. Both of these conditions are likely reactions to dizziness, rather than a cause, as open places don't have surfaces that can be used for support, or close visual referents. Treatment is usually best offered by a psychiatrist.

5. **Visual vertigo.** In this condition, the feelings of imbalance and dizziness are induced by the movement of visual scenes, such as watching television or watching traffic. Visual vertigo is common in both patients with vestibular (inner ear) disorder and patients with anxiety problems. The treatment may involve treating anxiety with medication and dizziness with vestibular rehabilitation therapy.

6. **Post-traumatic stress syndrome.** This is a severe anxiety disorder that can develop following a very stressful event such as the death of close friend, or a severe physical, sexual, or psychological injury that is usually beyond one's ability to cope with. This can cause dizziness with or without a spinning sensation. Treatment is usually offered by a psychiatrist.

7. **Malingering.** Malingering is possible in patients where there is a lack of physical findings or test abnormalities and a secondary gain factor. There is usually a pending litigation or compensation claim. It is also common in children who wish to avoid going to school. It is difficult to diagnose and probably best to refer to a psychiatrist for management.

ADVICE FOR HEALTH-CARE PROFESSIONALS

1. It is important to diagnose the underlying psychological condition appropriately as some patient may need a referral to a psychiatrist. Anxiety and depression are the commonest underlying causes.
2. The treatment of psychogenic dizziness may involve anti-depressants and rehabilitation therapy.
3. Good doctor-patient relationship will help in managing these patients, as accusing patients of faking illness may results in violence, and litigation against the doctor.
4. One way to communicate with the malingering patient is to suggest that all symptoms do not fit into the objective criteria of the diagnosis, allowing the person to rethink.
5. The clinicians may have to rely on special neuropsychological test for the diagnosis

ADVICE FOR PATIENTS & CARERS

1. Psychogenic dizziness requires treatment like any other illness, so there should not be any embarrassment in being diagnosed with this condition.
2. There is no quick treatment for this condition. Patients often require treatment for months before seeing any improvement

SUMMARY

Psychogenic dizziness is a common cause of chronic dizziness. Anxiety and depression are among the common causes. The patients usually have vague and elusive symptoms, with no physical findings and objective test abnormalities. The success of treating malingering behaviour is dependent on reward of the malingering behaviour. Patients may have to be referred to a psychiatrist for definitive treatment. The definitive treatment is usually provided by a GP, psychiatrist and a physical therapist.

FURTHER READING

1. Pollak L, Klein, C, Rafael S, Vera, K, Rabey, JM. "Anxiety in the first attack of vertigo". Otolaryngol Head Neck Surg. 2003 Jun; 128(6):829-34.
2. Afzelius, L, Henriksson, NG, Wahlgren, L. "Vertigo and dizziness of functional origin". Laryngoscope 1980; 90:649 656.
3. Baloh, RW, Sloane, PD and Honrubia, V: "Quantitative vestibular function testing in elderly patients with dizziness". Ear, Nose and Throat 1989; 68:935 939.
4. Belal, A, Glorig, A. "Disequilibrium of aging (presbyastasis)". J Laryngol Otol 1986; 100:1037 41.

Chapter 17

Acoustic neuroma (AN)

Case study: A sixty-six-year-old Parkinson's disease sufferer visited his GP with balance problems that had worsened over the months. A full physical examination did not reveal any new problems, apart from complete loss of hearing on right side, which was confirmed after a specific hearing test. A brain scan organised by the GP revealed a large acoustic neuroma tumour in the brain (at cerebello-pontine angle). He was immediately referred to a neurosurgeon for treatment. The size of the tumour was reduced by surgery and he made an uneventful recovery. His balance improved after the operation, but he required a hearing aid for his deafness.

INTRODUCTION

Acoustic neuroma is a non-cancerous tumour arising from the lining (myelin sheath) of the nerve concerned with hearing and balance (vestbulocochlear nerve). It is a slow-growing tumour and usually does not spread to other parts of the brain. AN represents about 8% of total brain tumours in adults and is rare in children. The median age of diagnosis is 50 years. It can be present in both ears in people suffering from neurofibromatosis type 2-NF2 (a genetic condition affecting the nerves). If diagnosed early and with appropriate treatment, most people can live a normal life.

CAUSES & SYMPTOMS

The precise cause of AN is not clear. However, the following are potential risk factors:

- Prolonged exposure to loud noise or music
- Genetic factors. Approximately 10 % of people with NF2 will have bilateral AN

- People with a history of parathyroid tumours may have increased risk of developing AN

This tumour is very slow-growing, so there may not be any symptoms in the first few years of appearance. However, the most common symptoms include:

- Deafness
- Tinnitus
- Dizziness (which may also be caused by infection or inner ear crystals)
- Facial symptoms such as numbness, pain, and tingling etc are present in about 25% of patients, especially those with large tumours. This is likely a pressure effect on the neighboring nerve (the trigeminal nerve).
- Headache is not a common symptom; however an enlarged tumour can cause an increase in pressure on the brain and may lead to headaches.

DIAGNOSIS & TREATMENT

The diagnosis is usually made after careful history, examination, a hearing test and an MRI scan (magnetic resonance image) of the brain. An audiogram (hearing test) is a good screening test for AN, as it is positive in almost 95% of the cases.

AN are non-cancerous tumours that can be treated successfully in the majority of patients. However, there is about a 5% chance of recurrence, particularly in people with NF2.

1. Surgery can remove the tumour in over 95% of cases. This technique depends upon the size of the tumour. Complications include deafness and facial weakness due to damage to the surrounding structures.
2. Radiotherapy will help in shrinking or completely removing the tumour. It can be used in isolation and after surgery if a small tumour is left behind.

3. Stereotactic surgery is a relatively new technique that delivers a large single dose of radiation to the precise local area of the tumour. This will cause less damage to the surrounding structures.

ADVICE FOR HEALTH-CARE PROFESSIONALS:

1. Any patients with dizziness and deafness would need a hearing test (audiogram). If there is unilateral deafness, then the patient would need an urgent referral to an ear, nose and throat specialist for a possible brain scan.
2. AN surgery is performed by ENT surgeons and neurosurgeons, so check your local arrangements.

ADVICE FOR PATIENTS & CARERS:

1. Stereotactic surgery does not involve any cutting and stitching, and has claimed the greatest success in reducing the tumour size.
2. Further information can be obtained from the British Acoustic Neuroma Association (www.bana.co.uk).

SUMMARY

AN is a slow-growing benign brain tumour that takes several years to produce symptoms. Deafness is the commonest symptom, followed by tinnitus and dizziness. An MRI scan of the brain is the test of choice for the diagnosis. Surgery is occasionally performed to relieve the symptoms.

FURTHER READING

1. Propp, JM, McCarthy, BJ, Davies, FG, Preston-Martin, S. "Descriptive epidemiology of vestibular schwannoma". Neuro Oncol 2006; 8:1
2. Eldridge, R, Parry, D. "Vestibular schwannoma (acoustic neuroma)". Consensus development conference Neurosurgery 1992; 30:962

3. Matthies, C, Samii, M. "Management of 1,000 vestibular schwannoma (acoustic neuro: clinical presentation". Neurosurgery 1997; 40:1
4. Edwards, CG, Schwartzbaum, JA, Lonn, S, et al. "Exposure to loud nosie and risk of acoustic neuroma". Am J Epidemiol 2006; 163:327

Chapter 18

Dizziness and air travel

Case study: A fifty-three-year old female flew weekly for work, and occasionally experienced some dizziness with spinning sensation (vertigo) after flying. These symptoms usually made her life difficult for at least a week, and recovery sometimes took up to four months. Following an examination and review of her history, she was diagnosed as suffering from benign paroxysmal positional vertigo. She was advised to avoid reclining her seat during travel, and was asked to undertake home exercises to alleviate any residual symptoms, which typically disappeared within a few days.

INTRODUCTION

Every year, millions of people fly from one place to other both on short and long haul flights without much of a problem. However, dizziness is one of the commonest risks to health encountered during air travel. If you have organised an airline flight, then it is important to understand the risks associated with flying and how you can manage these risk safely without interruption to your journey.

Some people have unreasonable apprehension about flying when they have dizziness and balance problems. They are usually fearful that their problem may get worse. Air travel may induce motion sickness leading to dizziness.

These symptoms may be exacerbated on small planes, which have unpressurised cabins.

RECOMMENDATIONS FOR FLYING WITH EAR PROBLEMS:

1. Perilymph fistula (Inner ear condition): Flying may worsen symptoms and alternative transport should be considered.

2. Mal de Debarquement: Avoid flying where possible or plan for short flights and/or a stopover en route.
3. Benign Paroxysmal Positional Vertigo: Usually OK to fly, although temporary dizziness may be experienced, especially if seats are reclined.
4. Labyrinthitis or vestibular neuritis: Usually OK to fly.
5. Menière's disease: Usually OK to fly but pressure fluctuations may exacerbate symptoms.
6. Ear drum perforations: Usually OK to fly.
7. Simple "cold" with associated blocked nose: Avoid flying where possible if the symptoms are bad.
8. Psychogenic dizziness: Usually OK to fly.
9. Acoustic neuroma. Usually OK to fly
10. Dizziness in multiple sclerosis and Parkinson's disease: Usually OK to fly.

ADVICE FOR HEALTH-CARE PROFESSIONALS:

1. Nasal drops (xylometazoline hcl) can be prescribed or purchased over the counter for relieving "cold" symptoms (blocked nose).
2. Cinnarizine tablets can be prescribed or purchased over the counter for relieving symptoms of dizziness.
3. Steroid nasal spray taken for a few days prior to travel may reduce the effect of allergy symptoms.
4. A low dose of diazepam is useful if there is associated anxiety
5. Grommet insertion. A grommet is a small ventilation tube, usually inserted in the eardrum after an operation. It is mostly used in children with glue ears. However in adults, this can be used to avoid pressure fluctuations between the middle and external ear. It is very occasionally required for this purpose due to associated complications such as infection and bleeding.

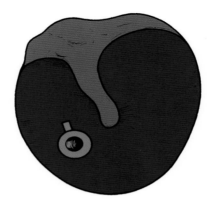

Grommet inserted antero-inferiorly

Fig 18.0

A grommet (ventilation tube) in the eardrum.

ADVICE FOR PATIENTS:

1. Individuals suffering from a common cold should avoid flying with a blocked nose. If this is not possible, then try to keep the eustachian tube open at take off and prior to landing to combat changes in cabin pressure. The eustachian tubes are narrow channels that connect the middle ear with the throat; they help to equalise the pressure. The eustachian tube can be opened by simply swallowing or chewing gum, and small children are encouraged to drink juice, water or milk intermittently.
2. Decongestant nose drops or spray e.g. xylometazoline 0.1% in adults, and 0.05% in children three to four times per day may help by opening up the nasal passages. It is available in pharmacies without prescription.
3. Some antihistamine tablets e.g. cinnarizine are available in pharmacies without prescription. They can be taken an hour before getting on the plane. These may help to manage pressure fluctuations by keeping the eustachian tube open.

4. Avoid sudden head movements that make your dizziness symptoms worse for about 1-2 days after flight.
5. Use two pillows at night for 2-3 days after flying to prevent dizziness.
6. Earplugs have become popular among frequent flyers, and there has been some anecdotal evidence that they help in reducing earache and dizziness following travel.

SUMMARY

Air travel is one of the commonest modes of travel worldwide. Mostly it does not cause any problems. However, millions of people either avoid flying or suffer from ill effects afterwards. With a good understanding of dizziness and balance problems caused by inner ear conditions, and with the help of appropriate advice, you can enjoy the flight.

FURTHER READING

1. Sen A, Al-Deleamy, LS, Kendiril, TM. "Benign paroxysmal positional vertigo in airline pilots". Aviat Space Environ Med 2007 Nov; 78(11):1060-3
2. Hain, TC. http://www.dizziness-and-balance.com. 16 Feb 2011

Chapter 19

Exercise-induced dizziness

Case study: A 35-year-old physiotherapist attended the Dizzyclear clinic, reporting severe vertigo while swimming. She had recently started an intense exercise program to remain fit and to reduce her weight. She was so fearful of these episodes coming back that she stopped swimming completely. After a four-week history of her symptoms and an examination she was diagnosed with Benign Paroxysmal Positional Vertigo (BPPV). She was treated in the clinic with Epley's manoeuvre, and after a few days of home exercises, her symptoms resolved and she was able to resume her swimming.

INTRODUCTION

Physical activity involves major muscle groups in performing daily activities, such as climbing stairs, walking, or shopping. Exercise involves an activity to maintain or improve physical fitness. Millions of people around the world are involved in physical activity every day. Physical fitness is defined as an ability to carry out daily tasks with energy and without excessive fatigue. Feelings of nausea and vertigo during workouts can be frustrating. This can happen occasionally after strenuous exercise, but may also happen after moderate exercise. In some individuals the exercises in which the head tips backwards, such as swimming, can mobilise the "crystals" in the inner ear (semicircular canals) causing dizziness symptoms. Most of the underlying causes for exercise-induced dizziness are simple and easily treatable.

Some of the common causes of dizziness during exercise include (please refer to the earlier chapters regarding management options):

1. Dizziness caused by inner ear problems:
- BPPV (most common)
- Perilymph fistula

2. Dizziness caused by neck problems:
- Arthritis of the neck
- Cervical cord compression

3. Dizziness caused by disease in the brain or spinal cord:
- Chiari malformation
- Superior canal dehiscence

4. Dizziness caused by blood pressure fluctuations:
- Postural hypotension
- High blood pressure during weight training

5. Dizziness caused by underlying diseases:
- Migraine
- Multiple sclerosis
- Heart rate and rhythm problems e.g. bradycardia, abnormal (ectopic) beats
- Medication side effects e.g. beta-blockers
- Viral infections

6. Dizziness caused by various physical activities:
- High impact e.g. during rugby, football leading to head injury
- Swimming

ADVICE FOR HEALTH-CARE PROFESSIONALS:

1) Postural hypotension may require altering medications.
2) A serious undiagnosed underlying cardiac condition (cardiomyopathy) can present with dizziness during physical activity

ADVICE FOR PATIENTS

1) If you have a known medical problem, such as a heart condition, blackouts, or seizures, then you should consult your doctor before starting regular workouts, as all of these conditions can lead to dizziness.

2) Keep well hydrated during a workout, as dehydration can cause nausea and dizziness.
3) Low blood sugar can also lead to dizziness; so make sure you have taken enough calories at least two hours before exercise.
4) A "head rush" feeling can happen due to a sudden drop in blood pressure. If any particular exercise is creating this feeling, try and perform it slowly. If it does not get better within one week, seek urgent medical advice.
5) Gradually build up your level of exercise severity, as progressing too quickly can cause nausea and dizziness.

SUMMARY

Exercise-induced dizziness is not a common problem. It may be present in some individuals and may cause interruption in regular exercise routine. Most of the causes are simple and easily treatable. However, occasionally this dizziness may be caused by underlying heart problems. If the dizziness does not improve and is interrupting your exercise, then you must get help from your GP initially.

FURTHER READING

1. Paffenbarger RS, Jr, Hyde, RT, Wing, AL, et al. "The association of changes in physical-activity level and other lifestyle characteristics with mortality among men". N Engl J Med 1993; 328:538
2. Haskell, WL, Lee, IM, Pate, RR, et al. "Physical activity and public health: updated recommendation for adults from the American College of Sports Medicine and the American Heart Association". Circulation 2007; 116:1081

Chapter 20

Dizziness and sex

Case study: A thirty-seven-year old man was referred by his GP to the Dizzyclear clinic. During consultation, he mentioned that his sex life has been seriously affected due to vertigo episodes during sexual activity. He described his symptoms as the room spinning, and feelings of nausea, whilst lying on his back during sexual activity. After an examination, he was diagnosed with benign paroxysmal positional vertigo (BPPV). A home Epley's manoeuvre was suggested as a remedy, and he was also advised to use two pillows while lying on his back. Three months following his visit to the doctor, his symptoms were completely resolved, with no recurrences during sexual activity.

INTRODUCTION

Embarrassment may prevent many people discussing dizziness during sexual activity, and it is mostly discussed as a corollary to other complaints. Some people are concerned that this may represent a psychological problem and that is not worth discussing. However, in most cases, the underlying cause is not serious and a simple treatment may resolve the symptoms.

CAUSES & SYMPTOMS

- Benign paroxysmal positional vertigo: This is the commonest cause of dizziness during a sexual encounter. Vertigo symptoms start after changing the position of the head, for example when lying flat on the bed without pillows, or when turning the head towards the left or right side. Epley's manoeuvre and using two pillows under the head at night can successfully relieve the symptoms.
- Anxiety and other psychiatric conditions: There may be an underlying anxiety about sexual activity that can present itself

as dizziness. The symptoms can last for a few hours and may improve with time. If it is recurrent, then it is possible that certain medications like diazepam may be required.

- Heart problems: During sexual activity there is an adrenaline rush, and people with underlying heart problems such as angina or dysrrhthmias (irregular heartbeat) can develop dizziness. This is a less common cause of dizziness.
- Medication side effects: Certain medications, such as beta-blockers, can reduce the blood pressure and may contribute to dizziness, particularly after getting up quickly. Viagra, which improves erectile dysfunction, can also cause dizziness, as can antihistamines, which are usually given for allergy treatment.
- Other less common causes include dehydration, overheating, arthritis in the neck, eye problems, particularly in the dark, tiredness, or prolonged breath holding during ejaculation, which can increase stress and lead to a migraine. Very rarely, a small bleed or even a tumour in the brain can cause similar symptoms.

DIAGNOSIS & TREATMENT

The diagnosis is usually made by a thorough history and examination and without any tests. Mostly the treatment involves home exercises and modification of position such as using pillows under the head during a sexual encounter. In addition, keeping well hydrated and being well rested can reduce stress. Some patients may need special tests such as a brain scan to exclude causes like a brain tumour or bleeding.

ADVICE FOR HEALTH-CARE PROFESSIONALS:

1. It is often difficult to get information about dizziness induced by sex. Therefore it is important for clinicians to explore this possibility of sex-induced dizziness.
2. Most medications given for dizziness can suppress sexual desire, so it is best to avoid medications and try home exercises, if possible.

3. Most performance-enhancing drugs, such as Viagra, can cause dizziness.

ADVICE FOR PATIENTS:

1. Simple measures can improve symptoms of dizziness during sexual activity like rehydration, getting enough rest, reducing stress, and a good and healthy diet.
2. Performance-enhancing medications bought on the internet may cause dizziness. If you need these drugs, then you must consult your GP or buy them from reputable health-care shops.
3. Most causes of dizziness caused by sexual activity are easily treatable, so do not hesitate to ask for advice from a health-care professional.

SUMMARY

Dizziness can happen during sexual activity. Mostly the cause is easily identified and treated. Occasionally it may represent an underlying serious problem; so if the symptoms do not get better with home exercises, contact your family doctor.

Chapter 21

Dizziness treatment using complementary and alternative medicine

Case study: A thirty-five year old started car sharing for work, travelling as a passenger on three days, and driving on the other two days of the week. He noticed that whilst travelling as a passenger, he would be nauseous, dizzy and had vomited on a few occasions. His close friend advised him to drink ginger tea half an hour before travelling. This remedy improved his symptoms significantly and he was able to complete the journey without significant nausea and dizziness.

INTRODUCTION

A growing number of doctors in the UK are turning to homeopathy and herbalism as an alternative to conventional medicine. Using natural remedies has been shown to alleviate many ailments, such as some skin conditions, dizziness, chronic joint and muscle pain, and anxiety disorders, where traditional medicine may have had little effect.

Plants and their derivatives have been used as medicine for healing purposes for many centuries and in all major cultures throughout the world. Since 1990, there has been as much as a 10-fold increase in the use of complementary and alternative medicine treatments. Some people believe that this is a natural way of healing ailments; some wrongly believe that this method of treatment is free of side effects. People are often persuaded by family members, or the media, to try these medications. There are a large number of medications sold that claim to treat dizziness. However, the following two are the most popular.

GINKGO BILOBA

This is one of the oldest types of trees still found in Korea, China, France and the United States. The leaves of this tree are used for medical treatment. Ginkgo is believed to improve circulation to the brain, which in turn improves its functions. It may be beneficial in treating the following conditions:

- Dizziness
- Short term memory
- Tinnitus
- Poor peripheral circulation

Ginkgo can cause an increased risk of bleeding due to its anti-platelet and antithrombotic properties. It can react with other medications, such as warfarin and aspirin, and may result in spontaneous bleeding.

GINGER

Ginger has been used for centuries for treating motion sickness, particularly in sailors. It is available in capsule or tablet form and can provide relief for the following symptoms:

- Nausea
- Vomiting, in pregnancy, after chemotherapy and in post-operative conditions
- Motion sickness
- Anxiety
- Cold and flu symptoms

WARNING

There is the potential for herbal medications to interact with medication prescribed by clinicians, as well as over-the-counter medications. You can ask your GP or pharmacist for advice. One useful online tool to check for specific interactions between natural and other medications is Lexi-interact (http://www.lexi.com).

ADVICE FOR HEALTH-CARE PROFESSIONALS:

1. Ask patients about the use of complementary and alternative medications. Most patients may not disclose to their doctor unless asked. This should be recorded as a part of medication history in the patient notes.
2. You may consider herb-drug interaction when prescribing conventional medicines.
3. Clinicians should try to establish the underlying reason for using complementary and herbal medications. Some alternative medications are sold for the prevention of heart diseases. Some people with a strong family history of heart disease may use them "to protect the heart." If there is a strong family history of heart disease, then the appropriate risk can be calculated and reassurance and evidence-based medications can be offered.
4. In the UK, further information can be obtained from NHS Direct (www.nhsdirect.nhs.uk) and NICE (National Institute of Clinical Excellence (http://www.nice.org.uk). This provides information on the latest treatments and information about drugs and supplements.
5. There is very limited robust data to suggest the safe use of alternative and complementary medication in pregnancy and breastfeeding, infants, the elderly, and in post-operative patients.

ADVICE FOR PATIENTS & CARERS:

1. Always mention to your doctor any use of alternative or complementary medications, so that appropriate help and medication can be offered.
2. It is advisable to buy all complementary medications from an alternative care practitioner registered with UK institute for complementary and natural medicine.

3. If you develop any side effects, ensure that these are reported to your GP, as there may be a solution to reverse the side effects.
4. Do not take gingko if you have any sort of bleeding disorder.
5. Ginger should not be used in people with gallstones, as it increases the production of bile and may cause gallstone conditions worse.

SUMMARY

Alternative and complementary medications are used widely throughout the world for various illnesses. Their popularity has grown significantly in the last 20 years. Most people wrongly believe that they are free of side effects. There is some evidence to suggest that Gingko Biloba and ginger help with dizziness symptoms. However, great care should be used and you should contact your doctor if you develop any side effects.

FURTHER READING

1. Le Bars, PL, Katz, MM, Berman, N, et al. "A Placebo controlled, double blind randomised trial of an extract of gingko biloba for dementia". North American EDb Study group. JAMA 1997; 278:1327
2. www.naturaldatabase.com
3. www.naturalstandard.com
4. www.consumerlab.com

Chapter 22

Vestibular rehabilitation therapy (VRT)

Case study: A 50-year-old policeman was punched in the face by a drunken adolescent while on duty at night. A hospital emergency department treated him for facial swelling, vomiting, and dizziness. A scan of the head and neck was performed, but came back negative. As a precaution, the patient was kept in hospital overnight for observation. He returned to his GP after about three months complaining of dizziness, which was especially bad during self-defense training. He was referred to an ear, nose and throat specialist. Following an examination, his care was transferred to a physiotherapist for vestibular rehabilitation, which relieved the symptoms after five sessions. The symptoms were nonexistent after six weeks.

INTRODUCTION

VRT is an exercise-based programme that is used to manage dizziness or balance problems caused by damage to the balance organ of the inner ear (the vestibular system). Most VRT exercises involve head movement, as these movements are needed for the recovery of the affected vestibular system. VRT has been highly successful for most adults and children with disorders of the vestibular or central balance system. The success of VRT is dependent on the patient's motivation, good general physical and mental health, the integrity of other sensory systems, and a relatively young age (less than 75). The main benefits of VRT include a reduction in falls, less feelings of dizziness and anxiety, and an improvement in balance, co-ordination and mobility. The common exercises used in VRT programme include Cooksey-Cawthorne exercises, Gaze Stabilisation exercises, a Canalolith repositioning manoeuvre such as Epley's maneouvre and Brandt Daroff's home exercises.

Who would benefit from VRT?

Most causes of dizziness involving vestibule (inner ear) would benefit from vestibular rehabilitation:

- BPPV (benign paroxysmal positional vertigo)
- Vestibular neuritis
- Acoustic neuroma
- Meniere's disease
- Perilymphatic fistula
- Post-traumatic vertigo
- Disequilibrium caused by aging
- Inner ear operations
- Psychogenic vertigo

Dizziness not involving the vestibule (inner ear) would be unlikely to benefit from VRT:

- Drop in blood pressure when standing from sitting position (postural hypotension)
- Vertigo associated with migraine
- Transient ischemic attack (stroke)

WHY IS VRT NEEDED?

The brain is dependent on information from the inner ear regarding balance, but when the inner ear is damaged with disease or injury, the brain can no longer rely on this information. This can result in dizziness, vertigo, balance problems, and other related symptoms. The brain has the ability to recover and compensate for this illness. This is called vestibular compensation, and typically occurs within a few weeks.

WARNING

After the brain has successfully compensated this balance problem, the symptoms can recur if there is a sudden interruption in daily activities

– for example after an operation, or following illness. The brain can "forget" what it has learned, a process called "decompensation". This process appears to be reversible if a sufferer undertakes a course of home exercise. However, some people may need referral to a clinic if the symptoms do not improve. This may suggest further damage to the vestibule (inner ear).

WHO WILL PROVIDE VRT?

Successful VRT involves a multidisciplinary team of health-care providers with experience in treating patients with balance problems. This team usually includes a doctor with experience in the assessment and treatment of balance disorders (usually an ear, nose and throat specialist or a neurologist), and a therapist (physiotherapist or other physical therapist) trained in balance testing and vestibular therapy.

ADVICE FOR HEALTH-CARE PROFESSIONALS:

1. Once the diagnosis of vestibular disorder is made and one of the above conditions is recognised, VRT can be safely started at home. It is worth warning the patient that symptoms may temporarily worsen during the early stages of treatment.
2. The progress of rehabilitation should be checked through clinical assessment and various standard questionnaires, such as the dizziness handicap inventory and activies-specific confidence scale. Within a clinical setting, posturography, rotatory chair testing, active head rotation test, and an electronystagmogram (ENG) may be performed to measure the response to treatment.
3. On occasion, the patient may need a referral to a special clinic, particularly if the symptoms are severe or there is no improvement.

ADVICE FOR PATIENTS:

1. If you suffer from recurrent dizziness and have been assessed by a doctor before, then you may wish to start VRT at

home (e.g. Cooksey-Cawthorne exercises, Gaze stabilisation exercises and at-home Epley's manoeuvre).

2. Sporting activities that you may help you in balance training include:
   - Basketball, tennis, table tennis, volleyball
   - Tai chi
   - Walking
   - Yoga
   - Nintendo-Wii, Playstation Move and X-Box Kinect
   - Trampolining
3. You may wish to contact your GP for a referral to physiotherapy or rehabilitation department for these exercises.
4. There are some private balance clinics where you can self-refer for assessment and rehabilitation.

VRT PROGRAMME:

A progressive programme of VRT exercise can be beneficial to a well-motivated patient. These exercises begin at a low skill level before progressing on to more complex stages and to complete recovery.

There are numerous exercises available; however the following are commonly used to treat a variety of balance problems. Please refer to subsequent chapters in the book for further details of these exercises.

- Cooksey-Cawthorne exercises (chapter 24)
- Gaze Stabilization exercises (chapter 25)
- Canalolith repositioning manoeuvre such as Epley's manoeuvre and Brandt Baroff's home exercises (chapter 27 & 28)

SUMMARY:

VRT is a programme of exercises that help to improve dizziness and balance problems mainly caused by inner ear dysfunction. This can be done preferably in a clinic, under supervision, or at home. These exercises do not provide a "quick fix" to the problem, but with patience, motivation and persistence, most patients recover fully.

REFERENCES:

1. Horak, FB et al. "Effects of vestibular rehabilitation on dizziness and imbalance". Otol HNS 1992:106-175
2. Fujini, A and others. "Vestibular training for benign paroxysmal positional vertigo". Arch Otolaryngol HNS 1994:120:497
3. Walker, C, Brouwer B, Culhan, EG. "Use of visual feedback in retraining balance following acute stroke". Physical Therapy, 80,9,200-

Part 2
Understanding Vertigo and its Management

Self management of vertigo using Dizzyclear pillow

VERTIGO

1. Worse with movements
2. "Spinning" sensation
3. Short duration
4. Nausea or vomiting

Perform Dix Halpike maneouvre

Positive

Negative

If the bad side "left or right ear" is known

If "bad ear" is not known

Consult your GP, you may need vestibular rehabilitation therapy (VRT)

Perform home Epley`s manoeuvre

Perform Brandt Daroff exercises

If no significant improvement within 3 weeks consult your GP

Khalid Bashir

Chapter 23

Benign Paroxysmal
Positional Vertigo (BPPV)

Case study: A 45-year-old university lecturer was suffering from recurrent bouts of vertigo associated with certain head movements for several years. His work was affected, as during his lectures, he used to get vertigo, especially on turning around. He tried various medications without much relief. He was diagnosed with BBPV. Epley's repositioning manoeuvre was carried out in the Dizzyclear clinic, and the patient's symptoms were completely resolved. He was also given home exercises in case it recurs again. The symptoms did recur again, but he was able to treat himself with home exercises such as home Epley's repositioning manoeuvre and Brandt Daroff home exercises.

INTRODUCTION

Benign paroxysmal positional vertigo is the most common cause of dizziness. It is a type of giddiness induced by various positions of the head. It is thought to be caused by tiny fragments or debris (calcium carbonate) in the posterior semi-circular canal derived from the inner ear structure called the utricle. Often referred to as "ear rocks", in the past, this debris was called "otoconia". In many cases, this condition clears away on its own after several weeks. A simple treatment of moving the head into various positions over a few minutes and home exercises can resolve the symptoms. This treatment uses gravity to move the debris away from where it is causing symptoms.

BPPV is a common condition of the inner ear and is a frequent cause of dizziness among outpatient clinic visitors. It is widespread in all ages, but much more common in elderly people.

Benign means that it is not a serious condition. (The symptoms may be troublesome, but the underlying cause is not serious.)

Paroxysmal means the recurrence of certain symptoms.

Positional means the symptoms of vertigo are produced by certain head positions.

Vertigo is dizziness with a spinning sensation. There is often an association of feeling sick or actual vomiting.

CAUSES & SYMPTOMS

There is no single cause responsible for this condition. However causes can be attributed about 40% of the time and include:

- Head injury
- Spontaneous degeneration of the labyrinth
- Post-viral illness (viral neuronitis)
- Complication of middle ear (stapes) surgery
- Chronic middle-ear disease (infection)

RISK FACTORS

- Age: onset is most common between 40 and 60
- More common in women (M:F 1:2)
- Meniere's disease (co-diagnosis in up to 30%)
- Migraine
- There is usually a history of injury, infection, tiredness, recent travel and nausea

ACTIVITIES THAT BRING ON BPPV:

The activities that produce these symptoms vary in different people. However, they are almost always triggered by a change in position of head with respect to gravity:

- When the head is tipped backwards to look up. Hence, it is also called "top shelf vertigo".
- When the head is tilted backwards on a hairdresser's shampoo bowl, it brings on the symptoms of "parlor vertigo".

- Repeated attacks of vertigo are often experienced after certain head movements (such as those entailed in rolling over in bed, lying down, sitting up quickly, leaning forward or turning the head in a horizontal plane).

SYMPTOMS

The symptoms of BPPV are intermittent and usually last for a few minutes. This can happen many times in a day. BPPV can disappear completely for some time, but can recur again.

Recurrent vertigo attacks are of sudden onset and usually last less than a minute.

Symptoms are typically worse in the mornings, and can include nausea and vomiting, lightheadedness, balance problems, and blurred vision, along with a sense of vertigo.

Usually one ear is worse. Patients often volunteer that symptoms are worse when the head is tilted to one particular side.

DIAGNOSIS & TREATMENT

BPPV can be diagnosed from a careful look at the patient's past history and from an examination, without the need for further tests. The Dix-Halpike manoeuvre (see below) can confidently diagnose BPPV. In some cases, the sign and symptoms are not very clear. Hence, your doctor may order further tests, such as electronystagmography (ENG) or viedonystagmography (VNG). These tests detect abnormal eye movements (nystagmus) caused by inner ear dysfunction if the head is put in various positions or when your balance organ in the ear is stimulated with water. It uses electrodes on the face, around the eyes, or video to record the results. Scans of the brain, including magnetic resonance imaging (MRI) or computerized tomogram (CT) may also be used to detect other serious conditions in the brain, such as tumours or bleeding.

DIX-HALPIKE MANOEUVRE

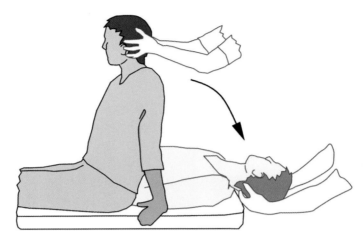

Fig 23.1

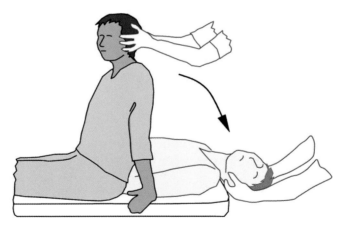

Fig 23.2

The Dix-Halpike manoeuvre is done by extending the neck and then rotating the head towards one side first. In this position, bring the patient down with their head hanging down over the edge of the bed. The patient is kept in this position for about thirty seconds. If the test is positive, after a short pause you may see the nystagmus (involuntary movement of eye ball). This is associated with intense feelings of vertigo. It usually wears off in 20-30 seconds. When the nystagmus stops, the patient sits up and symptoms can recur, with the nystagmus beating in the opposite direction. The test is repeated on the opposite side if the first is negative.

Treatment

1. Epley's manoeuvre by the doctor or at home by the patient (see chapter 27)
2. Brandt-Daroff home exercise (see chapter 28)

ADVICE FOR HEALTH-CARE PROFESSIONALS

1. The Dix-Halpike test can confidently diagnose BPPV.
2. Epley's manoeuvre can be done safely in clinic or GP surgery.
3. Instructions for an at-home Epley's manoeuvre and Brant-Daroff home exercises can be given from the clinic.
4. An anti-emetic e.g. stemetil, meclezine can be given for 1-2 days if nausea or vomiting is a real problem.
5. Sleeping with 2 or 3 pillows will help in preventing vertigo in the morning

ADVICE FOR PATIENTS

1. If after reading this information, you feel that you are suffering from BPPV, an at-home Epley's manoeuvre would be very useful in relieving your symptoms.
2. At night, use at least two pillows if possible.
3. Sit down if you feel dizzy.
4. If you get up at night, use good lighting.
5. Try and use a stick for walking if the dizziness is bad.
6. Before you see a specialist, keep a diary of your symptoms, including aggravating and relieving factors. Write down any questions that you would like to ask the doctor.
7. Bring a friend with you for a doctor's appointment who can take you home, as some patients' vertigo symptoms can get worse for a few hours after treatment.

WHAT CAN I DO IF THE MANOEUVRES ARE UNSUCCESSFUL OR SYMPTOMS HAVE RECURRED?

In author's experience, the above manoeuvres are successful in over 95% of patients, provided the diagnosis is made correctly. Some common causes of failure of manoeuvre treatment include:

- The diagnosis may have been wrong – for instance, the patient may have been suffering from central positional vertigo (causes in the brain), bilateral BPPV and rarely anterior canal BPPV.
- The patient may have not performed the manouevres correctly at home.
- BPPV can recur after successful treatment by exercises in about 30% of patients. Most recurrences (80%) occur within the first year of treatment. These recurrences can be treated at home with a home Epley's manoeuvre and Brant-Daroff exercises.
- In the remaining patients, "habituation" exercises (vestibular rehabilitation training) may relieve the symptoms completely. However, if the symptoms are intolerable in spite of the above exercises, then definitive surgical management may offer a permanent cure.

SURGICAL TREATMENT

Surgery is reserved for the most resistant and severe cases. All procedures carry the risk of damaging the nerve. The various procedures include:

1. Posterior canal plugging. This is the simplest of the procedures, in which the posterior semi-circular canal is surgically plugged. This prevents the loose particles from causing vertigo. This procedure has been reported to be successful in over 90% of cases, with less hearing loss.
2. Singular (Posterior ampullary) and Vestibular Neurectomy. This involves surgically cutting off the nerve that goes to part of the balance organ. It carries with it the same risk as brain

surgery, as well as the possibility of injury to the hearing apparatus and the nerve to the face.
3. Labyrinthectomy. This is quite a destructive procedure that involves removing the entire balance organ. It can be done chemically or surgically, and usually causes permanent deafness on the affected side.

SUMMARY:

BPPV is an extremely common cause of dizziness. It can be easily diagnosed and safely treated at home. The majority of patients get better with home exercises. It can recur again and usually responds well to home exercises. A minority of patients do require further treatment.

FURTHER READING:

1. Lee, NH, Ban, JH, Lee KC, Kim, SM. "Benign paroxysmal positional vertigo secondary to inner ear disease". Otolaryngol Head Neck Surg 2010; 143:413
2. Hain, TC. http://www.dizziness-and-hearing.com. 27 Oct 2010
3. Simhardi, S, Panda N, Raghunathan M. "Efficacy of particle repositioning maneuver in BPPV: a prospective study". Am. J. Otolaryngol. 2003; 24(6): 355-60
4. Epley, JM. "The canalith repositioning procedure: for treatment of benign paroxysmal positional vertigo". Otolaryngol. Head Neck surg. 1992; 107(3): 399-404
5. Semont, T, Freyss, G, Vitte E. "Curing BPPV with a liberatory maneuver". Adv. Otorhinolaryngol. 1988; 42: 290-293
6. Brandt, T, Daroff, RB. "Physical therapy for benign paroxysmal positional vertigo". Arch. Otolathinolaryngol. 1980; 106(8):484-5
7. Dix, Mr., Hallpike, CS. "The pathology, symptomatology and diagnosis of certain common disorders of the vestibular system". Ann Otol Rhinol Laryngol 1952; 61:987

Chapter 24

Cooksey-Cawthorne Exercises (CCE)

The purpose of these exercises is to improve the brain's ability to compensate for dizziness caused by a problem in one or both inner ears. They were first used to treat service personnel in the 1940s who suffered from balance problems during the war. These exercises may make dizziness symptoms worse initially. The more frequently dizziness is induced, the more quickly the brain compensation mechanism is built up. In between the exercises, normal life should resume. An early return to work and participation in sports will help with rehabilitation.

The sooner the exercises are started, the quicker the chance of compensation. If tolerated, the exercises are started for five minutes at a time, four times daily (20 minutes per day), and gradually increased to an hour per day.

PLAN OF EXERCISES.

Perform the following scheme of exercises if it is safe to do so.
1. **Sitting position**
a) Eye movements up and down, then from side to side, while focusing on your finger at one foot away initially and then at three feet away from your face, repeat 10 times.

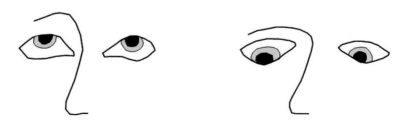

Figure 24.1a eye movement up/down

Cooksey-Cawthorne Exercises (CCE)

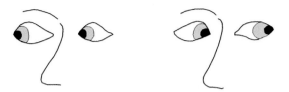

Figure 24.1a eye movement left/right

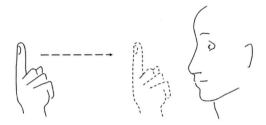

Figure 24.1a finger to eye

b) Head movements, initially with eyes open, then with eyes closed. Turn your head from side to side, and then nod up and down, repeat 10 times.

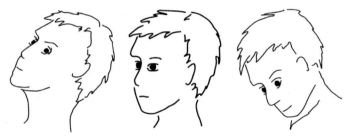

Figure 24.1b head move side to side, eyes open

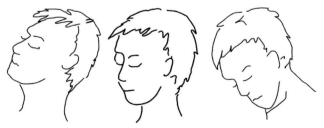

Figure 24.1b head move side to side, eyes closed

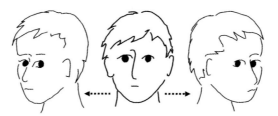

Figure 241b head nod, eyes open

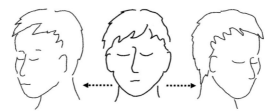

Figure 241b head nod, eyes closed

c) Shoulder shrugging and circling, repeat 10 times.

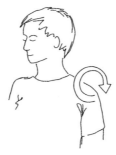

Figure 241c shoulder shrug

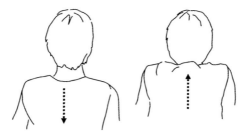

Figure 241c shoulder circling

d) Bend forward (if possible) to pick up objects from the ground, repeat10 times.

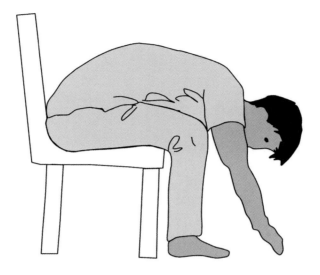

Figure 241d bend forward when sitting

2. Standing position
a) Eye, head and shoulder movements, as above.
b) Move from sitting position (if possible) to standing position with eyes open and then closed, repeat10 times each.

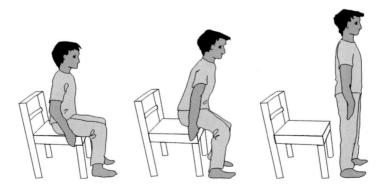

Figure24.2b sit to stand, eyes open

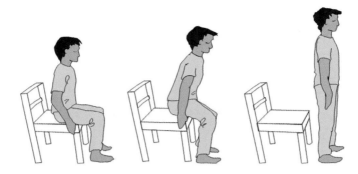

Figure24.2b sit to stand, eyes closed

c) Throw a ball from hand to hand above eye level and then under the knee, repeat 10 times each.

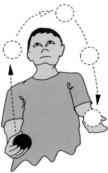

Figure24.2c throw ball over head

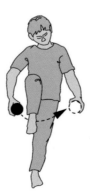

Figure24.2d throw ball under knee

3. **Walking**
a) Walk across the length of the room with eyes closed, and then open, repeat 10 times.

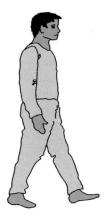

Figure24.3a walk along, eyes open

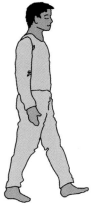

Figure24.3a walk along eyes closed

b) Go up and down stairs with eyes closed, and then open, repeat 10 times. If you live in a bungalow or a flat you can use a step ladder of 4-5 steps.

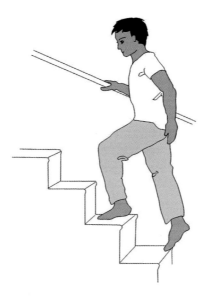

Figure24.3b walk up steps, eyes open

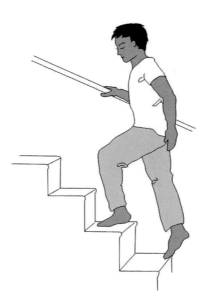

Figure24.3b walk up steps, eyes closed

c) Walk in a circle with someone standing in the middle of the circle. You throw a ball to this person who will return it back to you, repeat 10 times.

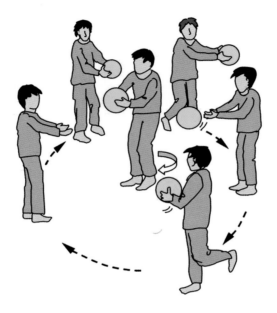

Figure24.3c walk in circle, throw/catch ball

SUMMARY

CCE are effective rehabilitation exercises. They can be done in the comfort of your own home. The most benefit is gained through regular exercises, and improvements are usually seen within six week to three months. In the beginning, the exercises may make dizziness symptoms worse.

Chapter 25

Gaze stabilisation exercises (GSE)

INTRODUCTION

If it is not possible to do CCE, (Chapter 24) due to severity of dizziness symptoms or some other disability you can start with GSE. GSE are particularly useful for chronic dizziness. The underlying cause of dizziness may not disappear, but the exercises teach the brain to adapt to this disabling condition. The aim of these exercises is to improve your ability to focus and also to improve vision on a fixed object when the head is moving. It is extremely useful to have a therapist supervising these exercises, at least in the beginning. Start with a simple task and progress to something more complex. These exercises should be done every day for about 30 minutes, preferably at various intervals, rather than all at once. The exercises can make you feel dizzy, particularly in the beginning, but if you start feeling sick, then you can stop for a day and restart the next day. If you stick with these exercises, the symptoms usually get better. In authors experience most patients do feel improvement with in six weeks of these exercises.

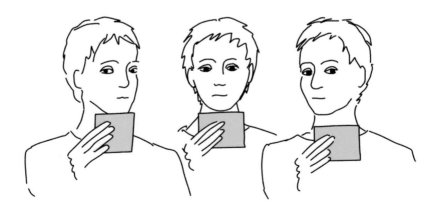

Figure 25.1

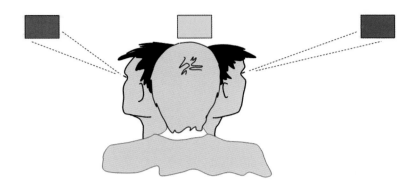

Figure 25.2

TECHNIQUE

1. **Head movement.** You can either sit on a chair or preferably stand up and hold an object – a credit card, for instance – in front of you at eye level. Slowly turn your head from side to side while your eyes remain focused on the object. Begin with one minute and, if tolerated, progress to two or more minutes. This should be repeated three times per day.

2. **Targets on the wall.** Place three targets on a wall, such as red, amber and green cards. These should be clearly visible at a distance of one metre initially, progressing up to three metres. One target should be in front; one on the extreme right and one on the extreme left. Either sitting on a chair or standing, move your head from left to right, looking briefly (less than a second) at each target. Initially, start with one minute, and then progress to two minutes. Initially, you should aim for 10 cycles per minute, gradually increasing to 20 cycles per minute. This should be repeated three times per day.

3. **Walking.** Repeat the above exercise moving your head from left to right whist walking back and forth, across a room for example. This is usually done once the above two exercises are confidently completed.

FURTHER READING

1. Herdman, SJ. "Role of vestibular adaptation in vestibular rehabilitation". Otolaryngol Head Neck Surg 1998;119: 49-54.
2. Herdman SJ, Schubert, MC, Tusa, RJ. "Role of central preprogramming in dynamic visual acuity with vestibular loss". Arch Otolaryngol Head Neck Surg 2001;127: 1205-10.
3. Hall, CD, Heusel-Gillig, L, Tusa, RJ, Herman, SJ. "Efficacy of gaze stability exercises in older adults with dizziness". J Neurl Phys Ther 2010 June: 34(2): 64-9.

Chapter 26

Dix-Halpike manoeuvre

The Dix-Halpike manoeuvre is performed to diagnose benign paroxysmal positional vertigo (BPPV). This test is usually done by a doctor in the clinic or GP surgery, however in the author's experience, it can also be performed at home using the Dizzyclear pillow. The patient is asked to sit on the bed and rotate the head towards the left side first (Fig 26.1). In this position, the patient is asked to move so that the head overhangs the Dizzyclear pillow. (Fig 26.2). The patient is kept in this position for about 30 seconds. If the test is positive, after a short pause, the vertigo symptoms may return and you may see the nystagmus (involuntary movement of the eye ball). It usually wears off in 20-30 seconds. When the nystagmus stops, the patient sits up and symptoms may recur with the nystagmus beating in the opposite direction. The test is repeated on the right side if the left is negative (Fig 26.3 and 26.4).

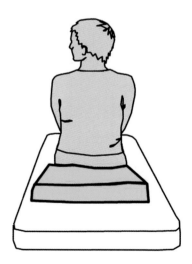

Figure 26.1 Sitting up and head turned to the left side

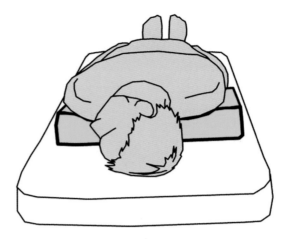

Figure 26.2 Lying on the back with head turned to the left at 45' and overhanging the Dizzyclear pillow.

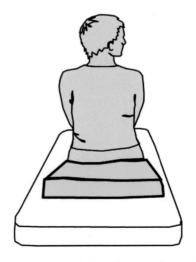

Figure 26.3 Sitting up and head turned to the right side

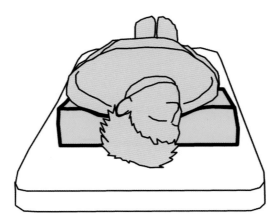

Figure 26.4 Lying on the back with head turned to the right at 45' and overhanging the Dizzyclear pillow.

Chapter 27

Modified Epley's manoeuvre (MEM)

Epley's manoeuvre was first described by Dr John Epley in 1980. There are many modifications to the original manoeuvre that are being used by different doctors and physiotherapists. The author has been using a modified Epley's manoeuvre since 1999, with excellent results. MEM is usually successful in relieving the symptoms of BPPV by moving the particles (crystals) out of the semi-circular canal. It is usually performed by an experienced clinician. However, if the diagnosis is clear, it can also be performed safely at home by using the Dizzyclear pillow. Each position lasts for an average of 30 seconds. We recommend three cycles each night, taking less than 15 minutes in total. At home, it needs to be done daily until symptoms completely resolve (usually within three weeks).

SCC stands for superior semicircular canal, while PCC stands for posterior semicircular canal and LCC stands for lateral or horizontal semicircular canal.

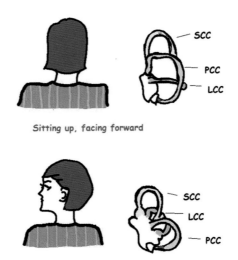

Sitting up, facing forward

Sitting up, facing left

Figure 27.1 Sitting up and then facing left

The following illustrations (Fig 27.1 - 27.2) show the movement of crystals in the inner ear along with various manoeuvres.

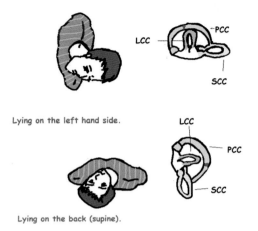

Lying on the left hand side.

Lying on the back (supine).

Figure 27.2 lying on left side, and then lying on the back

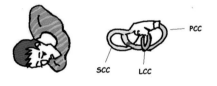

Lying on the right-hand side.

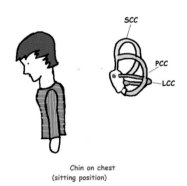

Chin on chest
(sitting position)

Figure 27.3 Lying on the right side, and then sitting up with chin on the chest

MEM ILLUSTRATIONS USING DIZZYCLEAR PILLOW

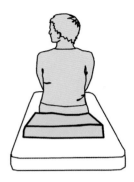

Figure 27.4 (a-e)
a. Sitting up and facing left side

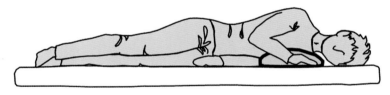

b. Lying on the left side with head overhanging the pillow

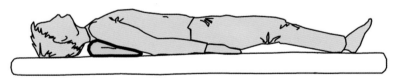

c. Lying on the back with head overhanging the pillow

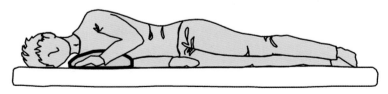

d. Lying on the right side with head overhanging the pillow

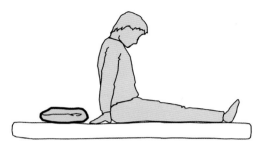

e. Sitting up with chin on chest

Followings illustrations will show a second technique of doing home Epley's manoeuvre. This is particularly useful if the patient has difficulty in rotating the whole body to either left or the right side. Start with head rotation to right if symptoms are bad on the right side, however if symptoms are worse on the left side start with head turning to the left side.

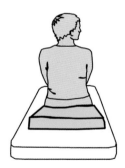

Figure 27.5 (a-e)
a. Sitting up and facing right

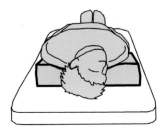

b. Lying on the back with head 45' to the right

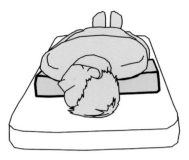

c. Lying on the back with head 45' to the left

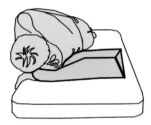

d. Rolling to the left with facing down

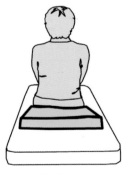

e. Sitting up

INSTRUCTIONS AFTER MEM

After the above manoeuvre, the following instructions should be followed to prevent a recurrence of vertigo symptoms. The symptoms usually recur during certain movements, such as tipping the head backwards, as this position will mobilise the crystals in the inner ear. These precautions are usually necessary for about 1-2 weeks after the treatment.

1. Immediately after the manoeuvre, wait for a few minutes before doing various activities.
2. Try and keep your head vertical and avoid movements or exercises that involve moving the head backwards such as cleaning the top shelf at home, neck exercises, etc.
3. Have a shower while standing and avoid bathing.
4. Avoid swimming.
5. Take extreme care while visiting the dentist, hair salon, or physiotherapist for back problems.
6. If eye drops are required, avoid bending your head backwards.
7. Use two or three pillows at night and avoid lying on the "bad side".

Chapter 28

Modified Brandt-Daroff Exercises (MBE)

MBE describe a series of exercises that are performed at home using your own bed and a Dizzyclear pillow. This is particularly useful when the "bad ear" is not clear. In the lying position, the head overhangs the pillow, as this position induces the most dizziness. The exercises are performed on average three cycles, three times per day for three weeks. It will take four positions to complete one cycle: sitting, lying on one side, sitting again, and lying on the other side. In the lying position, with the head overhanging the pillow, try and keep your eyes focused at the ceiling. Each position should last for about 30 seconds or until the vertigo symptoms subside, and should not last for more than one minute. Most people feel an improvement within one week of these exercises.

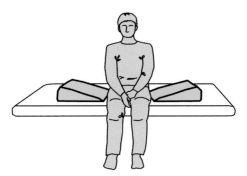

Figure 28.1 Sitting on the bed

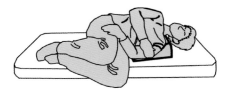

Figure 28.2 Lying on the left side with
head overhanging the pillow

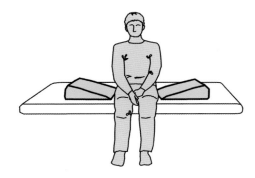

Figure 28.3 Sitting on the bed

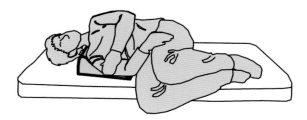

Figure 28.4 Lying on the right side with
head overhanging the pillow

SEMONT'S MANOEUVRE

The Semont's manoeuvre is performed to dislodge crystals to stop
the symptoms of vertigo. It takes about 10 minutes to complete
the treatment and is usually done by a doctor. This is only
mentioned for readers to understand this technique, however, the
author has not used this procedure for his patients. This may not
be suitable for the patients to use at home. The procedure is briefly
summarised below.

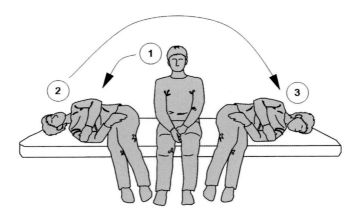

Figure 28.5

- While the patient is sitting straight up on the examination table bed, the head is turned away from the "bad side".
- The head is lowered to the side, causing vertigo. While lying down, the eyes look at the ceiling. This position is held for approximately 2-3 minutes.
- The patient is then quickly moved to the opposite side without stopping in the upright middle position. Again, this position lasts for 2-3 minutes.
- The patient will then be moved to sitting position, again for 2-3 minutes.

Chapter 29

Frequently asked questions

1) Is feeling dizzy the same as having vertigo?

   No. Vertigo is just one specific type of dizziness, which is usually caused by problems with the inner ear. You can feel dizzy without having vertigo symptoms. Dizziness, simply, means feelings of light-headedness or unsteadiness. Patients often feel dizzy before they faint. This can be secondary to a strong emotion, standing for a long time, or standing up too quickly from sitting position. Dizziness and fainting are very common and in most cases, not serious. However, if your symptoms are prolonged, then you should get in touch with your GP to discuss these issues. Other conditions can also make patients feel dizzy, for example, a problem with the rhythm of your heart, thyroid gland problems, side effects of some drugs, and other conditions, including problems within the brain.

2) How is balance controlled?

   Balance is controlled by the following three systems:

   - Inner ear (vestibular system)
   - Eyes (visual system)
   - Sensory receptors in the skin, muscles and joints maintain our balance when we stand or walk. This is known as proprioception – the body's ability to sense movement

3) Can I drive if I am diagnosed with benign paroxysmal positional vertigo (BPPV)?

   If the symptoms are bad, then you need to stop driving. If the symptoms are well controlled and you remain symptom-free, you can start driving again. In the UK, you can contact the DVLA for further advice. You may also contact your GP to discuss in more detail. Drivers with a group 2 licence for large goods vehicle and passenger-carrying vehicles need to be symptom-free for the duration of the journey in order to be eligible for driving.

4) Is BPPV an early sign of stroke?

Although some symptoms are similar to stroke symptoms, BPPV is not an early sign of stroke. A careful review of the patient's history and an examination will help in correctly diagnosing this condition. A simple manoeuvre can help to alleviate the symptoms.

5) I live alone; can I do these exercises on my own at home?

Most people can do home exercises in the comfort of their own home on the bed or on the floor. However, it may be useful if a friend or relative can assist with some exercises, especially during the early part of the treatment.

6) My dizziness is still no better in spite of having surgery to my inner ear (labyrinthectomy).

Most patients' dizziness takes time to recover following major operations. If the symptoms are no better within three months, then you should consider referral for vestibular rehabilitation therapy.

7) Which drugs potentially lead to hearing loss?
   1. Salicylates, such as aspirin
   2. Aminoglycosides (gentamicin, tobramycin, amikacin)
   3. Erythromycin (antibiotic)
   4. Cisplatin and related compounds (chemotherapy)
   5. Loop diuretics (furosemide, bumetanide)

8) I play contact sports, when can I go back to playing again?

Most dizziness symptoms usually resolve in one to three weeks of the treatment. When your symptoms have disappeared, you can go back to sports. If these symptoms of dizziness (BPPV) recur, performing the home Epley's manoeuvre can provide relief.

9) What is the Dizzyclear pillow?

The Dizzyclear pillow has been specially designed to diagnose and treat a type of dizziness (BPPV) in the comfort of your own

Frequently asked questions

home. Most suffers may be able to self diagnose by filling in an on-line Dizzyclear questionnaire.(www.dizzyclear.com).There are clear instructions provided along with the pillow to help patients in self-management.

10) Shall I do fewer activities to help with dizziness?
Inactivity will not help you to get better. The brain needs to be exposed to mismatching signals coming from two ears to help in compensation. Try and perform daily chores and participate in various exercises for dizziness. Do not suffer in silence – dizziness is extremely common. Try and talk to your GP to get early help.

11) I was told I would have to live with this dizziness for the rest of my life – is this true?
About 20 years ago, there used to be little in the way of treatment available for dizziness. Most patients used to get tablets for vertigo. At present, there are various methods available to treat dizziness very successfully. There have been recent advances in equipments for brain scans. Nowadays, most people with dizziness get successful treatment.

12) What is the commonest cause of dizziness?
In most patients, the underlying cause of dizziness is in the inner ear (the labyrinth). Hence, most treatments available are aimed at the inner ear, including medications and the vestibular rehabilitation programme.

13) I developed dizziness after an accident – can I claim compensation?
Dizziness can develop following an accident, particularly to the head and neck region. Most sufferers can get compensation for this condition following injury.

14) I developed stroke few months ago, can my dizziness be due to an inner ear problem?
Yes, dizziness with spinning sensation (BPPV) can develop along with other medical conditions such as stroke, Meniere's

disease, hypertension, head injury, epilepsy, or following meningitis. Most people can improve this dizziness with simple treatments at home.

15) Home treatment has successfully resolved my dizziness symptoms, but can they recur?
Yes, they can recur, but most people can self-treat at home with a modified Epley's manoeuvre, and/or Brant Daroff home exercises.

16) I am 32 weeks pregnant, and get dizzy spells when I lie down. Could this be due to an inner ear problem?
Yes, it is possible that you are suffering from BPPV and may benefit from home exercises. During the last three months of pregnancy, a lot of women also develop low blood pressure while lying down due to womb pressure on the blood flow to the heart (supine hypotension syndrome). This may also lead to dizziness. Lying on the left side may help to relieve these symptoms. This condition usually disappears when pregnancy is over.

17) I was diagnosed with labyrinthitis four months ago, but I am still suffering from dizziness. When will this get better?
Most people with viral labrynthitis get better within one week. However, occasionally, the recovery can take longer. It is important to get help from your GP, who may prescribe tablets and arrange referral to a therapist for vestibular rehabilitation.

18) Why do elderly people develop imbalance?
Healthy balance depends on a fully functioning vestibular system, normal vision, normal tracking, normal sensation, and pressure receptors (proprioception) in the lower extremities. People with impairments in each of these areas have multi-sensory imbalance. Usually, vision, visual tracking, and sensation in the feet become impaired with age. When coupled with any vestibular disorders or with a gradual age-related decline in vestibular function, multi-sensory imbalance occurs.

19) Are any treatments available for multi-sensory imbalance?
Firstly, any correctible deficiencies in vision or sensation should be treated. For example, cataract surgery can improve vision, and vitamin B12 supplementation can be provided for neuropathy due to a vitamin deficiency. Vestibular rehabilitation, including fall risk assessment, can help improve overall balance. During rehabilitation, assistive devices such as walking sticks and Zimmer frames can be used, and training can be given in their proper use.

20) What are other central causes of dizziness?
Trauma can result in direct brain injury or post-concussive syndrome. Other central processes include stroke, and multiple sclerosis. Tumours in the posterior fossa such as acoustic neuroma are also an important cause of dizziness and or hearing loss.

21) My mother suffers from dizziness. Will I get a similar problem?
It depends upon the type of dizziness. There is no scientific evidence to suggest that BPPV runs in families. However, Meniere's disease does have a genetic link.

22) What are the symptoms of a balance disorder?
When balance is impaired, you may feel that surroundings are spinning, and or you may fall to one side when you try to walk. Other symptoms include feelings of faintness, light-headedness, blurred vision, confusion, nausea, vomiting, inability to concentrate, faster heart rate, anxiety and panic attacks.

23) I was involved in an accident about 8 months ago, now I am getting vertigo symptoms. Could this be BPPV?
Yes, it is likely that you are suffering from BPPV. This injury may have been a trigger for crystals to move in the inner ear. It is common for people to develop symptoms weeks and months after the injury. The injury can be in the head and neck region or elsewhere, such as the ankle and foot region.

24) Is dizziness is sign of a serious disease?

Dizziness and vertigo are usually not a signs of serious disease. Dizziness symptoms are very common, particularly in elderly patients. Most of the sufferers can be treated very effectively by various exercises.

25) Where can I get further information about dizziness and balance problems?

The following links will help you to understand about dizziness and vertigo in more detail.

www.brainandspine.org.uk
www.balancenetwork.org
www.csp.org.uk
www.menieres.co.uk
www.vestibular.org
www.dizzyclear.com